STRETCHING
FOR A PAIN-FREE LIFE

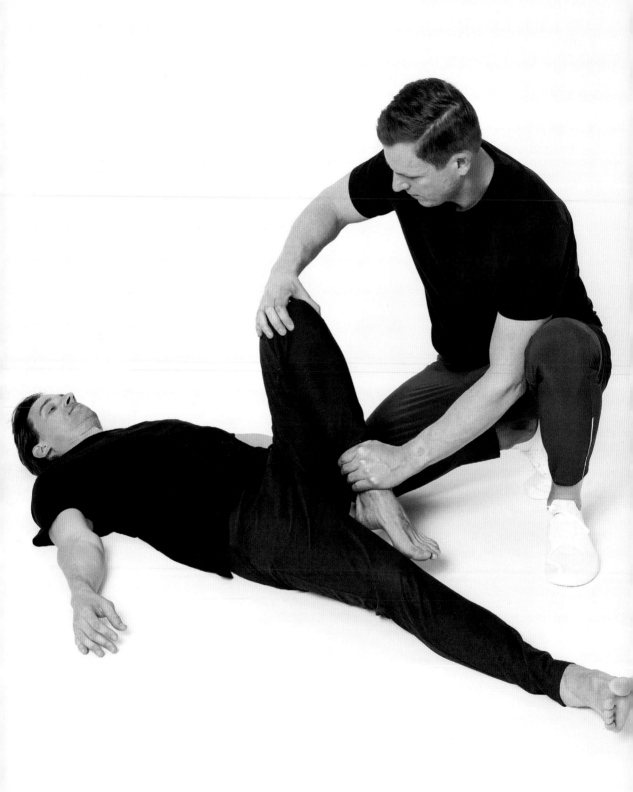

STRETCHING
FOR A PAIN-FREE LIFE

Simple At-Home Exercises to Solve
the Root Cause of Low Back, Neck, Knee,
Shoulder and Ankle Tension for Good

John Cybulski, DC and Bobby Riley, DC
Creators of The Anatomy of Therapy

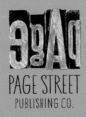

PAGE STREET
PUBLISHING CO.

PAGE STREET
PUBLISHING CO.

First published in 2023 by
Page Street Publishing Co.
27 Congress Street, Suite 1511
Salem, MA 01970
www.pagestreetpublishing.com

Distributed by Macmillan, sales in Canada by The Canadian Manda Group.

27   26   25   24   23   2   3   4   5

ISBN-13: 978-1-64567-962-2
ISBN-10: 1-64567-962-4

Library of Congress Control Number: 2022948026

Cover design by Katie Beasley for Page Street Publishing Co.
Book design by Molly Kate Young for Page Street Publishing Co.
Photography by Parker Thornton

Printed and bound in the United States of America

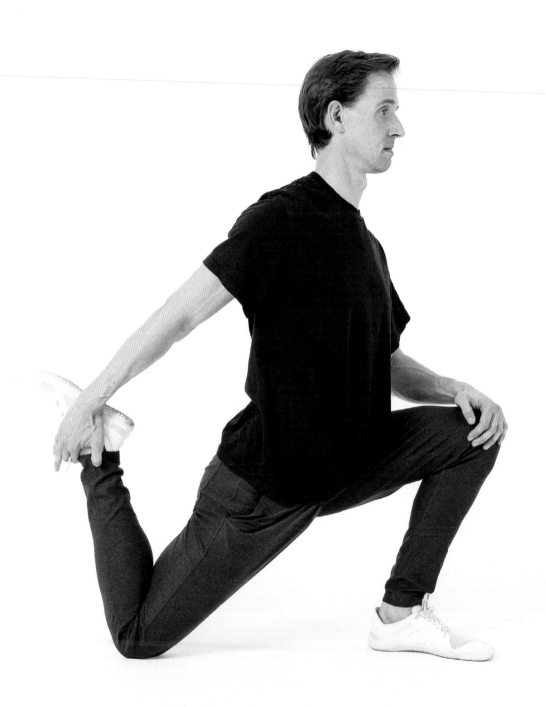

In memory of our friend, the late Dr. Stephen Offenburger

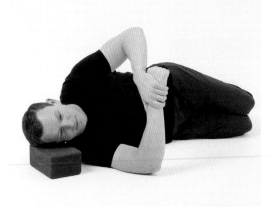

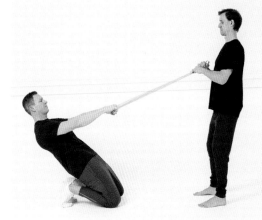

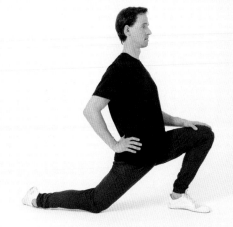

CONTENTS

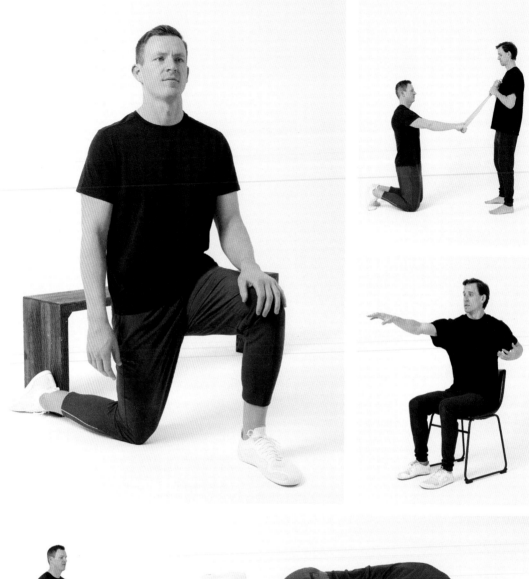
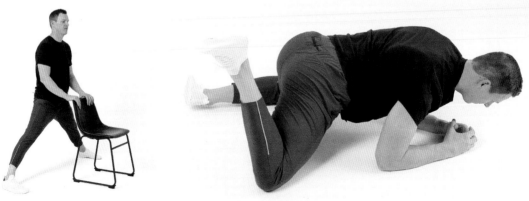

INTRODUCTION

There's a certain awe of the interconnectedness of the human body that has always intrigued me. Numbers make sense to certain people, but to me the manual bodywork involved in chiropractic (I graduated in 2010 with my doctorate) and how it worked to get people out of pain just clicked for me. As my practice developed, I learned the nuances of exercise and the impacts it had on pain. This became a useful skill as my practice emptied out during the pandemic. Everyone left the clinic and searched their phone for solutions. So, I decided to meet them there by starting an account on social media. After over 400 practice posts, our account went viral. Now over two million people follow us, and on any given month somewhere between two and ten million people see my exercises on their phones. It's been incredible to see that so many people have connected with something I am so passionate about. This book is another extension of that same passion. Thank you for taking the time to read this.

—John Cybulski

About 15 years ago, after an undergraduate degree and earning multiple national championships in track and field at the University of Wisconsin–La Crosse, I took the path toward a chiropractic doctorate. Near the end of my time there, I was fortunate to land an internship working primarily with NFL players and other professional athletes. My first foray into working on my own taught me two things: (1) Have skin in the game. Having people directly and solely depend on me for their recovery and rehabilitation gave me real impetus to get better, to learn more, and (2) Managing care is much more complicated than anyone had ever let on. I would have to set off on a lifelong journey to make sense of it all.

As any great chess player or hunter will attest, the real skill is in pattern recognition. I will be forever grateful to my chiropractic degree for incessantly reminding me that the body has the potential to heal itself, but the primary goal of schooling is to help you pass tests and memorize facts. Yet the real *truth*, if we may call it that, is in the patterns learned from the years spent hands-on with injured patients, professional athletes and friends. Humans are a lot more alike than they are different, and this book is an attempt at identifying the recurring patterns John and I have observed over our combined 20+ years. Almost 4 years ago we created a podcast to discuss and debate these patterns, to help new doctors, to aid listeners in their rehabilitation journey and to advance our own thinking as we sift through the complexities of the human body. Now with millions of followers, our brand, The Anatomy of Therapy, stands for this simple idea: Humans are the most adaptable creatures on Earth, and our potential to rebuild ourselves is unending.

—Bobby Riley

WHO IS THIS BOOK FOR?

This book is for anyone who wants to begin taking control of their present and future movement health. Whether you have something specific, like a nagging painful hip, or are smartly attempting to preserve your good hips into older age, this book can add some crucial value to your life. Let it serve as a guide for rebuilding yourself and maintaining your body. Because as you know, and probably do not reflect on enough, we have one body, and its components need to last quite a long time.

The prescriptions and plans within this book to help rebuild your body have been selected with the following issues in mind:

1. People have limited time.

2. People have limited energy.

3. People have limited equipment.

4. People have limited patience.

Time: You should be able to complete the exercises in each of The Stretches sections in this book in less than 10 minutes.

Energy: The stretches and movements are laid out in a progressive fashion so that you can begin with just movement 1 and stop after that, or just 1 and 2 and stop. Then eventually, you can progress to all the movements for that section once you are capable.

Equipment: There is no requirement for equipment in this book; therefore, each exercise can be done from almost anywhere. The use of any tools or small pieces of equipment (band, light weight, etc.) are strictly optional.

Patience: The plans within this book have been developed with the idea of seeing results quickly. One individual day may not seem to be moving the needle too much, but it will be the regular consistency that will hopefully show results within just a few weeks.

This book, therefore, is a useful tool for gauging when you need further professional help. If you are diligent and regularly partaking in the exercise sections that best fit your rehab demands and are not seeing results within a few weeks, then you can decide with much greater confidence to seek out the professional assistance of your local physical therapist, chiropractor, orthopedist or other relevant practitioner.

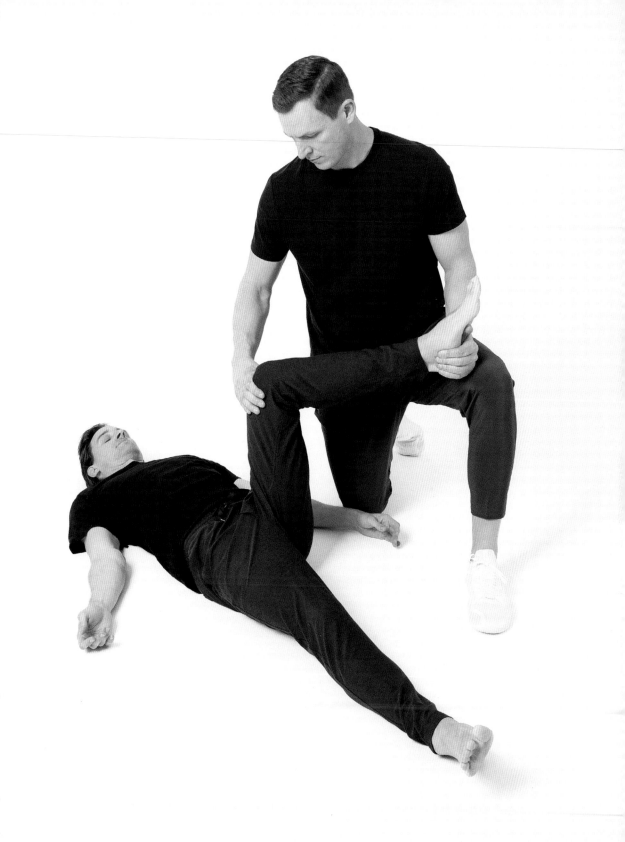

THE 80/20 PRINCIPLE

The primary challenge when writing a "rehab yourself" book for anyone or *everyone* is this: *Which information should be given in order to achieve the greatest probability of positive results with the lowest probability of risk?* Sounds easy enough, but I assure you it wasn't! The majority of the time spent creating this book was not in the outlining and writing or even rewriting, but rather in the deep analysis required to answer that single question.

The method by which we went about choosing the information in this book came from the 80/20 rule, also known as the Pareto Principle.

Vilfredo Pareto was an Italian economist who observed that 80 percent of all the land in Italy was owned by just 20 percent of its population, meanwhile also purportedly noticing that 80 percent of the fruits in his garden were born from 20 percent of the plants. Consequently, his observation came to be widely known as **the Pareto Principle, which states that roughly 80 percent of the consequences (outcomes) often come from only 20 percent of the input (effort).**

We attempted to apply the 80/20 rule to the best of our ability in this book. Using this principle, we have ultimately rephrased the question above to ask two better questions.

Based on 20+ years of combined clinical experience, the scientific literature and personal reflection, we instead ask the following:

1. What 20 percent of bodily issues are responsible for 80 percent of the disability, pain and dysfunction (consequences)? (For example, low back problems are much more responsible for medical costs and time out of work than finger pain or jaw dysfunction.)

2. What 20 percent of activities (effort: stretches, exercises, movements) will most likely be responsible for 80 percent of the improvements (outcomes: decreased pain, improved function) for any random reader in need of rehab help?

We, therefore, narrowed in on eight key areas of the body (the 20 percent) that we believe are most commonly responsible for the ailments and dysfunctions (the 80 percent) we see in the clinic or with our online followers.

And from there, in order to simplify this amazingly complex process for you, we pored over the endless options and varieties of stretches, exercises and helpful movements and reduced them to just the select few we believe will be the most effective and accessible activities. In other words, the movements (or the 20 percent) rendering the best results on average (the 80 percent).

THE EIGHT KEY AREAS OF THE BODY

It should go without saying, but needs reminding, that we are, all of us, the same. We are all *Homo sapiens*. On the surface it seems as though there are so many differences among us, but in the world of anatomy and physiology, this just isn't so. We are humans and we are plagued by human problems. We are not plagued with slug problems. (Who doesn't love salt?) Cheetahs are not plagued with chronic low back pain the last time I checked the Discovery Channel. (I am no feline expert, but I assume it isn't possible to sprint 70 miles per hour and tackle gazelles with debilitating sciatica.) Dogs have dog problems, nudibranchs have nudibranch problems and humans have human problems.

It should be no surprise, therefore, that when you look at data of populations from a plethora of different countries, they all show virtually the same complaints, and their health-care systems spend the most money on the same problems. We broke these omnipresent complaints down into the most common reasons why the areas of the body covered in this book (low back, shoulder, knee, etc.) are in pain or dysfunctional.

They are as follows:

1. Poor ankle and big toe mobility
2. Stiff, weak adductors (groin)
3. Tight torqued knees
4. Lack of internal rotation in the hips
5. Poor extension of the hips
6. A loss of thoracic rotation ability
7. Inadequate shoulder mobility and strength
8. A restricted and dysfunctional spine

If we can improve the movement quality and capacity of each of these individual eight areas, then we open the door to endless potential for them to work in harmony with each other. When this occurs, the body gains access to graceful, unhindered, pain-free movement, and your body should keep giving for years to come.

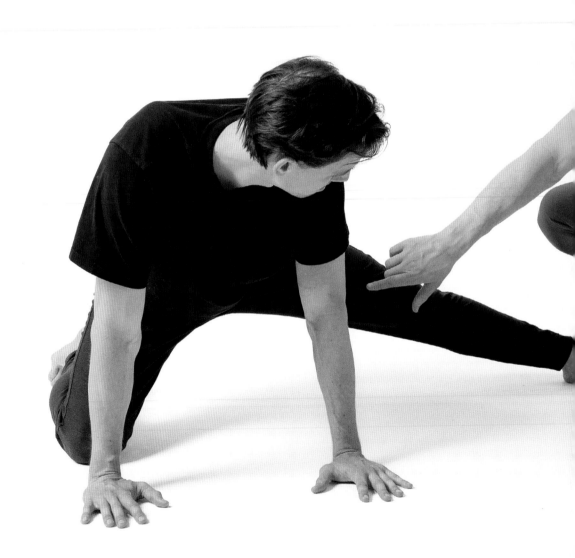

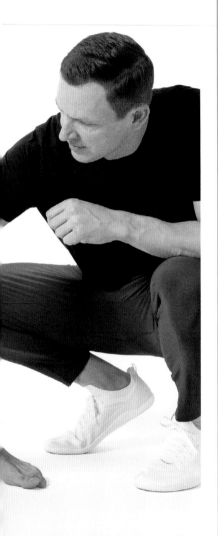

GOALIE GROIN

How Strong, Agile Adductors Are Game Changing

The groin region in most adults has the unfortunate circumstance of being overly tight and restricted and, additionally, weak and ineffective. This nasty combination often leads to a host of compensations and dysfunctions that can manifest themselves elsewhere in the body.

For example, a restricted, tight groin will prevent the pelvis from performing its natural rocking rhythm. If the pelvis cannot move forward or backward with ease, such motions as bending to touch one's toes or extending the hip fully, as in normal walking, become almost impossible tasks. Moreover, if the pelvis is "stuck" and the person can *still* touch their toes, that is equally worrisome because they have most likely adapted by loosening elsewhere beyond a desirable point. Restoring strength and flexibility to the groin (adductors) will improve our three-dimensional movement ability and secure the foundations for a strong core and robust breathing.

THE LOWDOWN ON THE GROIN

The groin, as we are defining it for the purposes of this chapter, consists of the adductor group. Named after the action of *adduction* (bringing your limb toward the midline of the body, e.g., squeezing a ball between your feet), this group of four muscles starts at the upper inside of the thigh and ends lower on the inside of the leg and knee.

Typically, when one considers the action of these groin muscles, they think only of side-to-side movement (frontal plane, see diagram below), such as a hockey goalie doing the splits or abruptly squeezing their leg pads together to block a late shot on the goal. But the groin muscle group is a robust, complex structure that helps assist the thigh up toward the chest and also assists in extending the thigh behind the body. In some positions the adductors rotate the thigh inward, and in other positions they can rotate it outward. Yes, the groin muscles attach to the leg and move it, but this muscle group also attaches to the pelvis and therefore moves *it*.

This is easy to understand when looking at a muscle like the biceps. The bicep bends the elbow, yes? It brings the hand toward the shoulder (bicep curl). Yes, but it also brings the shoulder toward the hand (pull-ups).

Easy-peasy, right? The good news is you do not need to fully understand the complexity of the groin. Try instead to simply understand a basic principle. *That principle is that most of us (the 80 percent) need to improve groin flexibility as well as groin strength.*

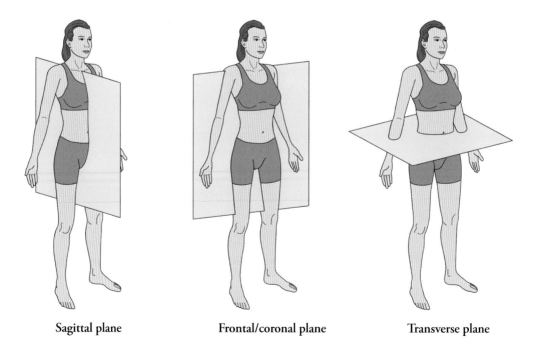

Sagittal plane   Frontal/coronal plane   Transverse plane

WHY YOUR GROIN IS SQUASHING YOUR POTENTIAL

As we have already alluded to, the group of muscles that make up the groin is vast and complex. When restricted, they can potentially prevent all directional movements of the hips, stunt pelvic motion and spine motion or create any combination of these.

Therefore, based on that alone, everyone should take the time and due diligence to at least explore the quality of their groin health. Especially those with knee problems, groin and pelvic issues, hip pain or low back pain. Improving the function of the groin complex isn't guaranteed to improve your pain, but it is almost guaranteed to improve how you move. And how you move is strongly correlated with how you feel!

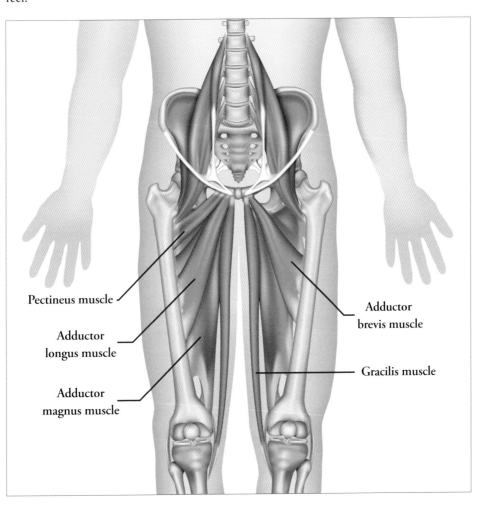

Pectineus muscle

Adductor longus muscle

Adductor magnus muscle

Adductor brevis muscle

Gracilis muscle

Why Adductors Are a Problem in Almost Everyone

When we are young, we play. Play is random and chaotic. We dance and flip and hang and tumble. The experience of playing sports like hockey, soccer and gymnastics is an ephemeral one, as we generally don't play them past our youth. We are young, our soft tissues are extensible and our joints are spacious. So why are groin problems in particular so problematic as we age? Well, because we replace guarding someone holding a basketball with walks around the block. We exchange our hockey skates for running shoes. We swap the balance beam for Jim Beam®.

Quick question: Which movement, crucial to most athletic activity, is rarely used in our daily lives and training routines as we age?

Short answer: Side to side. The frontal plane. In other words, moving your legs out to the side away from or toward the midline of your body.

The poor groin, previously a household name, an A-list celebrity, is now a washed-up has-been. Relegated to stabilizing the leg during marathons and manspreading on public transportation everywhere. Even sports like CrossFit®, which confers the title of "Fittest Person on Earth," have almost zero lateral (side-to-side) movements. We have to do what we can to keep those embers of what once was burning . . . or else pay the consequences.

WHY IT IS CRUCIAL TO MAINTAIN A STRONG GROIN

The original research and thinking behind adductor problems pointed toward inflexibility as the main issue. However, over time, more research has shed light on what might really be responsible for adductor health: strength or the lack thereof. One study (Engebretsen et al. *American Journal of Sports Medicine.* 2010. https://pubmed. ncbi.nlm.nih.gov/20699426/) showed subjects with weakness in the adductor muscle group were four times more likely to sustain an injury, while another study (Tyler et al. *American Journal of Sports Medicine.* 2001. https://pubmed.ncbi.nlm. nih.gov/11292035/) found that individuals were 17 times more likely to strain an adductor muscle if they had weak adductors.

In our clinical experience, we typically find it to be a double whammy in that the adductors are both extremely tight and restricting *and* at the same time suffer from being too weak. Now it does seem to be the case that tightness alone doesn't cause as many issues as weakness within the groin, but that tightness can be a silent killer for the functionality of other areas of the body, as previously mentioned. Therefore, we highly recommend addressing both factors with a slight emphasis on making sure you get that groin strong! That is what these following stretches aim to achieve; they build upon each other to address both issues.

THE STRETCHES

2

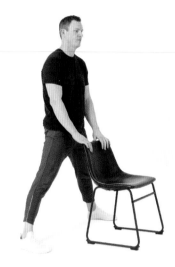

Standing Adductors–Contract-Relax (C-R)

In standing with the legs straight, we will be stretching and strengthening the long adductors that attach below the knee.

Step 1: Stand facing a wall with your hands placed lightly on the wall for balance. You could also use a chair or other piece of furniture.

Step 2: Begin by slowly spreading the legs apart until a light-to-medium stretch is felt in the inner groin.

Step 3: Once your stretch position is comfortably achieved, hold this position for 30 seconds.

5

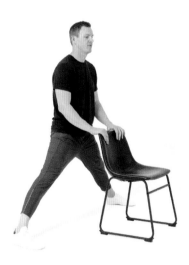

Step 4: Begin to contract (C) for 20 seconds into the floor, as if you were trying to bring your feet back together; you should feel your inner thighs engage.

Step 5: Relax (R) deeper into the stretch by carefully adjusting the feet farther apart (if safe and feels easy).

Step 6: Repeat steps 3 through 5 until no further progress can be made. Then do *not* hop out of the position quickly; rather, slowly and gently work the feet back together to a standing position.

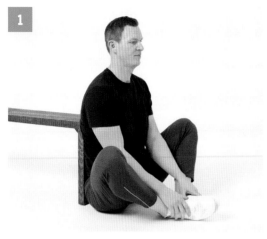

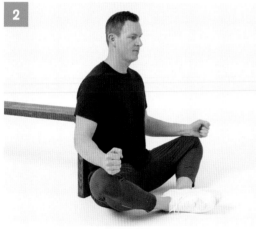

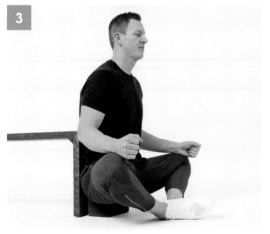

Tailor's Pose–Contract-Relax (C-R)

Also known as the butterfly stretch, this movement has the knees bent, which helps primarily to stretch and strengthen the short adductors that attach above the knee.

Step 1: Sit on the floor with your pelvis and back supported against a wall or steady object. Bend your knees, and place the bottoms of your feet together. Bring your feet close to your body comfortably.

Step 2: Using your hands, or resting light weights on your knees, gently push your knees toward the floor until you feel a medium stretch. Hold this position for 90 seconds.

Step 3: Using your hands, resist and prevent the knees from moving as they attempt to contract upward from the floor, and hold for 10 seconds.

Step 4: Relax and go further into the stretch if possible for 10 seconds.

Step 5: Repeat this process 5 to 10 times.

> **Note:** If sitting on the floor is too difficult, we recommend making the stretch easier by elevating the hips on a pillow or block.

Adductor Leg Lifts

The goal of this stretch is to load the adductors, directly promoting strength and resilience.

Step 1: Lie on your side with your bottom leg straight and your top leg crossed in front, with the knee bent and the foot flat on the floor.

Step 2: Engage your core first to stabilize your trunk.

Step 3: Raise your lower leg up off the ground as far as you can, and hold for 1 to 2 seconds. Slowly lower it to the ground.

Step 4: Repeat for 3 sets of 10 to 20 reps.

Step 5: Repeat on the other side (recommended even if the other side is pain-free).

Step 6: Once this becomes too easy, add weights to the foot or ankle.

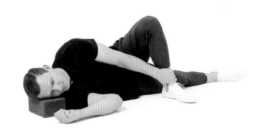

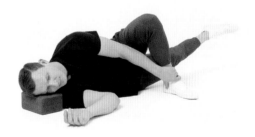

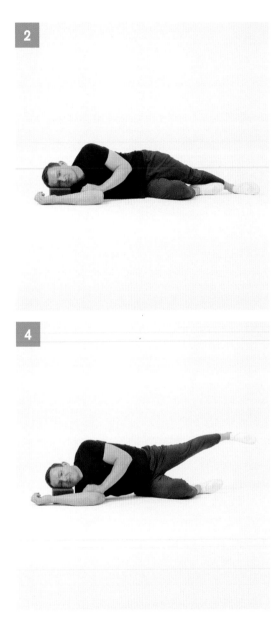

Abductor Leg Lifts

While this does not target the adductors directly, it acts to help round out hip strength and promote a stretch and relaxation of the groin muscles.

Step 1: Lying on your side, bend the bottom knee and hip to 90-degree angles.

Step 2: Rest the top leg's foot on the floor, and turn the hip just slightly into internal rotation by keeping the big toe on the floor but raising the heel off the floor.

Step 3: Engage the core to brace the torso.

Step 4: Holding the leg position, raise the top leg up as high as possible, and hold for 1 to 2 seconds.

Step 5: Slowly and under control lower the leg down, and touch the big toe back to the floor.

Step 6: Repeat for 3 sets of 10 to 20 reps, or 3 times as many as possible until you are eventually able to complete more than 10 reps per set.

Step 7: Repeat on the other side (recommended even if the other side is pain-free).

MOVING FORWARD

Let this theme of strength and flexibility stay with you. Having one without the other is a reliable path to future problems. This concept has been stressed here in the groin chapter because most readers will be missing both strength and flexibility there. But remember when assessing yourself to carry this concept into all areas of bodily movement.

As you develop strength and flexibility in the groin, compensations will reduce, and the body will begin working more harmoniously together. For ease of understanding, these vital areas are broken up into chapters, but remember, as each individual area gains capacity, the ability of the body to integrate all the separate areas into one collaborative body becomes increasingly possible.

"You're in pretty good shape for the shape you are in!"
–DR. SEUSS

"Your body has enough weight for you to be in perfect condition just working against yourself."
–JEAN-CLAUDE VAN DAMME

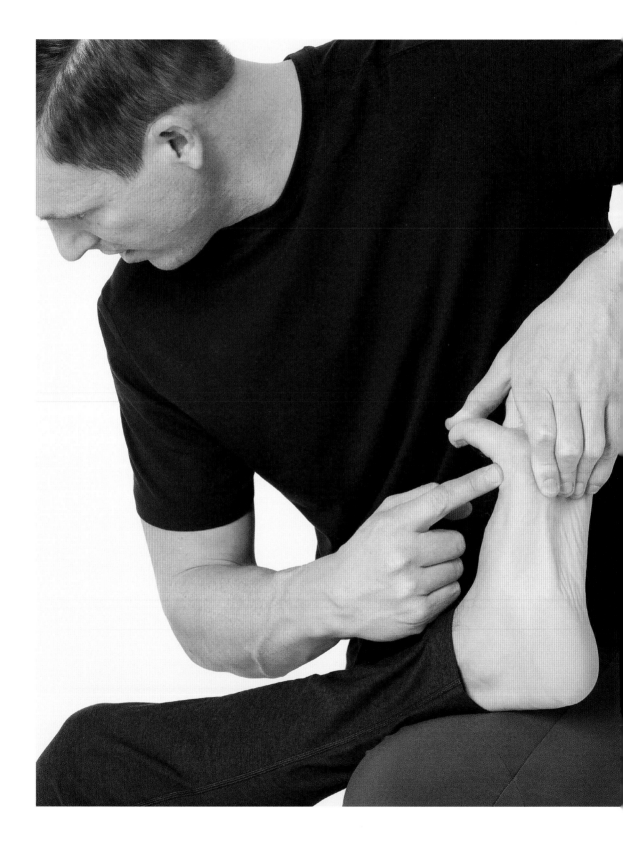

THE ANKLE ANGLE

Why Bad Ankles Make for Bad Knees, Hips and Low Backs

Your foot and ankle are made up of 28 bones, 32 joints and over 100 ligaments. There are so many things that can go wrong here, but fortunately you need to only be able to do a few things correctly to have a healthy foot and ankle. In this chapter you will learn why the foot and ankle get into trouble and how to get out of it.

The two major goals of the chapter will be to increase your overall range of motion and to regain control of the movement of your foot and ankle.

Learning to identify and correct problems in this area sets the foundation for the entire body. If the ankle is unstable, the knee will begin to compensate. If your ankle is over-pronating (rolling inward too much), it will cause the knee to twist inward. This is often the cause of pain on the inside of the knee. And if the knee is rotating inward, that means it's pulling the hip out and down. This dip in the hip not only tilts the spine to the side of the dip but also creates muscle imbalances along the way. But if we are able to cut the problem off at the base, we can begin to align things.

WHY YOU NEED TO ADDRESS THE ANKLE, TOE AND FOOT TOGETHER

Any change in the foot will change the way the entire leg works. This is most obvious if you get a shoe that changes the position of the foot because changing the slope of the foot, like when you wear a high heel or boot instead of being barefoot, changes the ankle's angle. The foot changes the ankle's angle, which in turn alters the knee position. Therefore, addressing this area as one piece begins to create harmony when everything works in concert.

WHAT IS OVER-PRONATION, AND HOW DOES IT CAUSE YOU PAIN?

Pronation is the inward twisting of the foot or forearm. Your hand pronates when you turn a door handle inward, and you *supinate* (the opposite) when you turn the handle outward, away from the body. The foot, ankle and toes can also roll inward and out. Ideally, their resting position is somewhere between rolled all the way out and rolled in. Being over-pronated is akin to a car with unbalanced tires. If you bump your wheels enough, you may notice the car "pulls" or doesn't naturally go straight. Being over-pronated pulls the body into an exposed position in which it is susceptible to countless compensations and eventual issues.

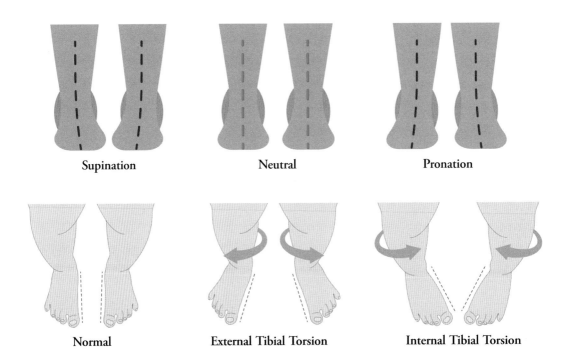

Supination   Neutral   Pronation

Normal   External Tibial Torsion   Internal Tibial Torsion

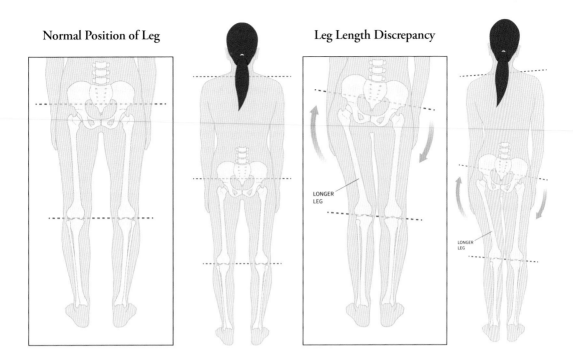

Normal Position of Leg

Leg Length Discrepancy

LONGER LEG

LONGER LEG

WHY ARE YOU FEELING PAIN IN YOUR FOOT?

Having limited range of motion and weakness are the two main causes of pain in the foot. Limited range of motion can occur via previous traumas, like broken bones or sprained ankles, but often foot pain is insidious (comes from "nowhere"). Having pain that "just started" without any traumatic incident is far more common than you think. These injuries are said to be the product of a series of dysfunctions. Compensations build up over time. These compensations lead to certain areas of your body becoming stronger and leave others weaker.

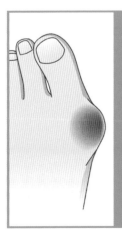

A Note on Bunions

The toughest toe trauma to tackle is bunions. Sometimes the bony reformation has gone too far, and only surgery will correct it, but I have also seen patients who were determined to not go the surgical route find success. Using a looped band around the two great (big) toes pulls the toes to the midline. This position needs to be held almost to exhaustion to reverse the outward pull of the toes. Being able to lift the toes into extension as they are being pulled toward each other is the second goal here, but the time spent pulling them straight is more important than doing repetitions.

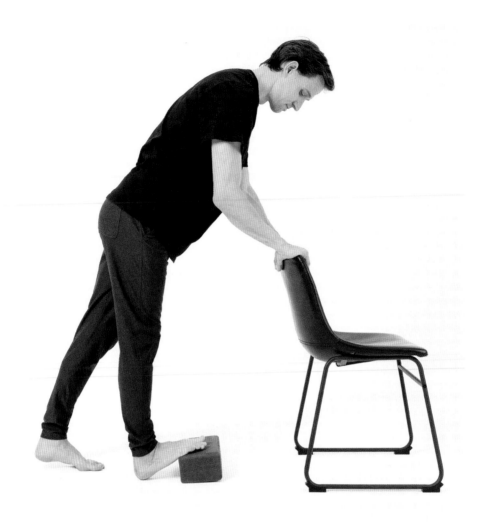

IMPROVING RANGE OF MOTION

The range of motion for your foot is like a swing. Its prime movement is forward and back. Improving the biggest range makes the biggest change. These two ranges are called *dorsiflexion* and *plantar flexion*. If you lack these ranges, your foot will have to rotate to make up for the lack. This is the "pulling" you want to avoid.

THE STRETCHES

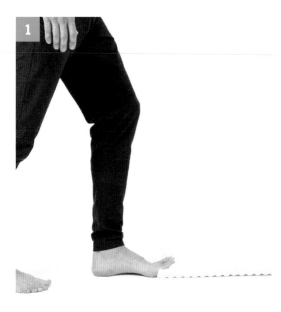

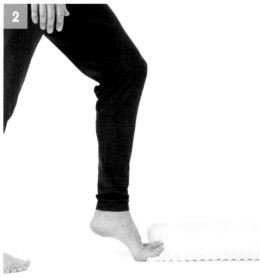

Great Toe Extension (Isolation)

Sometimes the great toe becomes so stiff and isolated you need to stretch it before you can integrate it with the rest of the body. While there is always some rotation at the great toe, you can make the most improvement by being able to fully bend and extend.

Step 1: Using a towel to prop up the great toe but leaving the ball of the foot on the ground, raise the heel and ankle off the ground then back down 15 to 25 times.

Step 2: Readjust the position of the great toe before adding pressure to the ball of the foot so that you notice a stretch on the arch of the foot.

Note: The primary movement is forward and backward, but feel free to shift the heel in or out to find a better stretch. The same goes for the next stretch.

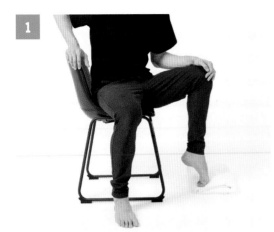

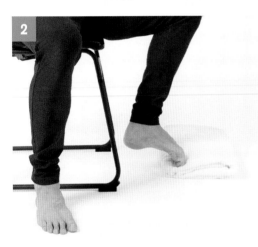

Great Toe Flexion (Isolation)

As the previous stretch focuses on extension, you must not neglect its opposite, flexion. If one is more difficult than the other, try to even them out by doing the one you are not as good at.

Step 1: Bend your great toe so the nail portion is on the ground with your foot pointed and over the toe.

Step 2: Lower your heel and ankle, but keep pressure on the front of the great toe, then bring the heel up and repeat 15 to 25 times.

Fixing Your Ankles—Dorsiflexion

Improving your range of motion will help most immediately, but connecting the great toe with your newfound range of motion is the key to long-term relief. The easiest way to improve dorsiflexion (or the forward motion of the foot) is by doing a calf stretch. The goal is to lengthen the muscles along the back of your lower leg.

Step 1: Place your foot at the edge of a stair, and allow your weight to drop back into the heel.

Step 2: Hold this tension in the back of the calf for at least 60 seconds, but try to build up to 3 minutes for the best results.

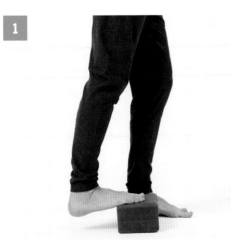

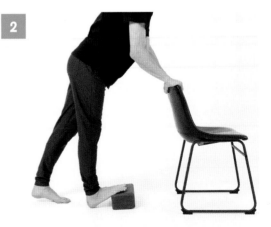

Fixing Your Ankles–Plantar Flexion

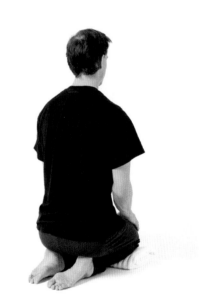

The easiest way to improve plantar flexion (or the backward motion of the foot) is to sit in the child's pose position. The goal here is the opposite of the dorsiflexion stretch. You are trying to lengthen the muscles along the front of the lower leg. This position may be very difficult at first, but this is only a sign that there's a lot of improvement to be made. Getting out of this position after you stretch can almost feel worse than when you started. This is very typical. With enough time and repetition you will find it gets easier. Try to stay in this position for at least 60 seconds, but build up to 5 minutes.

Step 1: Sitting on the shins and tops of your feet, allow your hips to put pressure on your heels, stretching the front of the ankle.

Step 2: Shift your hips to the left or right to balance the stretch.

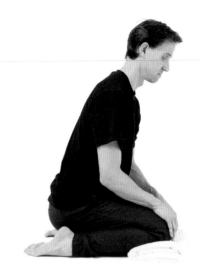

Step 3: Exit the position once you notice some tingling or numbness in your feet.

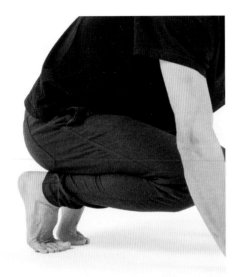

Adding in the Great Toe: Child's Pose and Toes

In order to restore balance to the foot and ankle, you will now alternate the position of the toes and ankle from the previous stretch. This position helps to stretch the plantar fascia with the added benefit of having a bit more tension from your bodyweight sitting on the heels. Lifting and lowering the knees 10 times will help to loosen the muscles on the bottom of the foot.

Step 1: Instead of pointing the foot straight, bend at the ankle and at the ball of the foot. Focus on putting your weight into the ball of the foot and great toe.

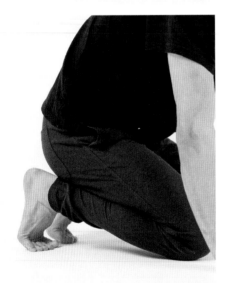

Adding in the Great Toe: Calf Un-Raises (Toe Raised)

Instead of focusing on the stretch of the big toe, you will now focus on slowly lowering the heel. This allows the calf and muscles of the bottom of the foot to learn to lengthen.

Step 1: Propping up the great toe, raise your heels (indirectly flexing the great toe), but focus on lowering the heel very slowly while maintaining pressure through the great toe and ball of the foot. Repeat 15 to 25 times.

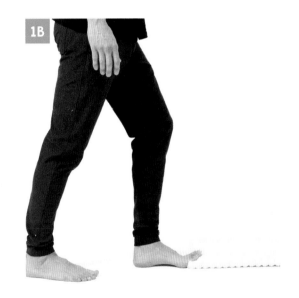

MOVING FORWARD

Progressing in these drills is a matter of time and attention. You also need to pay attention to the positions and areas of the body that are most sensitive. This is where you will be able to make the most change. Do not try to force these changes. Your body will adapt if you lean gently into the discomfort.

But as a wave is part of the whole of the ocean, it's important to avoid hyper-focusing on or isolating one problem area. In the coming chapters you will be learning how this all connects.

"Change before you have to."

–JACK WELCH

"True life is lived when tiny changes occur."

–LEO TOLSTOY

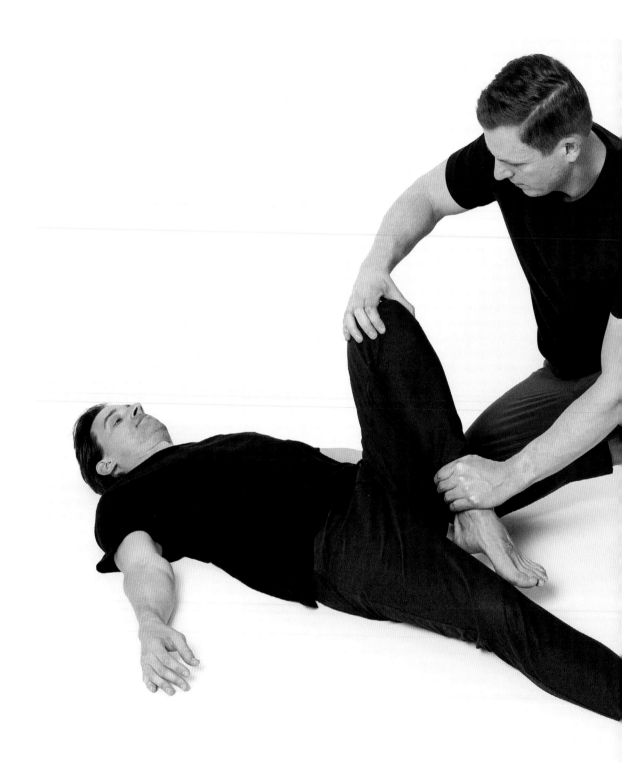

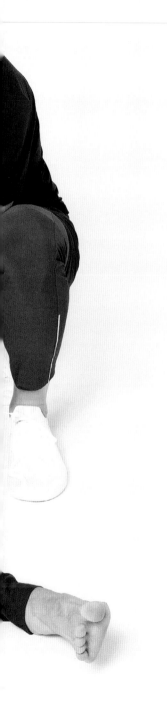

FREE THE KNEE

Why a Working Knee Is the Keystone for Movement

After a certain amount of time, having pain in the knee becomes triggered by certain patterns. These triggers happen when you move too much or move too little. Patterns that trigger pain can be bending or straightening the knee, sometimes with too much rotation. They could also come from problems in the joint, the muscle or a combination of both. The challenge in this chapter is in finding ways to unlearn harmful patterns, inverting the triggers and creating useful patterns to help you move.

There are three major functions of the knee, and in the coming pages you will learn how to address each in an effort to restore proper functionality.

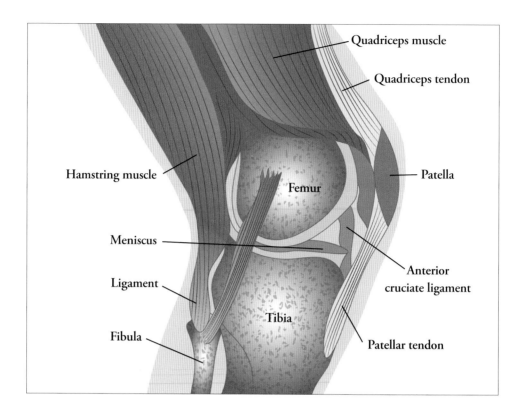

Quadriceps muscle
Quadriceps tendon
Hamstring muscle
Femur
Patella
Meniscus
Anterior cruciate ligament
Ligament
Tibia
Fibula
Patellar tendon

THE BIG THREE OF FREEING THE KNEE

A proper knee restoration can include many strategies, but the most essential categories to address are (1) controlling the joint, (2) controlling quad function and (3) practicing progressive loading strategies to increase your ability to absorb force. Often it takes only one of these three approaches to begin to restore normal function, but attacking the problem from all three angles gives you the best chance for recovery. Let's take a closer look at each of these three components.

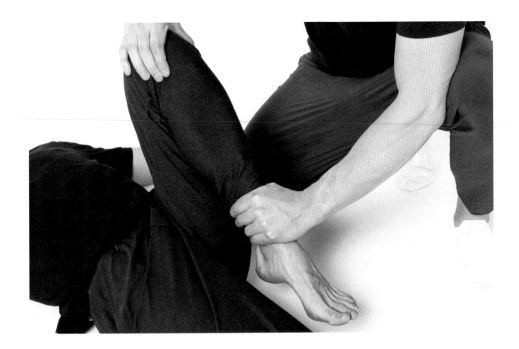

1: The Joint—Why the Knee Must Fully Bend

The joint space of the knee is mostly filled with *menisci* (like bumpers between your bones), which help keep bending and flexing the knee smooth. These surfaces slide and glide over each other until they don't. While it is the muscles' job to contract or relax to the forces placed on it, it's the joint's job to transfer that force.

Doctors test if you have enough joint space in the knee by checking *knee flexion*. Your ability to bend your knee (bringing the heel to the butt) is the first indicator of your knee's joint health. This becomes a problem when there is too much activity (trauma) or too little activity (being sedentary). These levels of activity often lead to developing unconscious patterns of movement that, though initially meant to protect the knee, will begin to limit it.

How Torque Is the Silent Killer of Healthy Knees

Your knee is a hinge joint, so it needs to flex forward and backward, not left or right. The *shear force*, or torque, on the knee that causes it to move left or right and not straight is the most common reason knees experience problems. Traumatic knee injuries always include rotation. Even with nontraumatic knee pain you will notice knees that are rolling in or out too easily. A common example of this is when you change directions quickly, like twisting to get in and out of your car. Once you notice it, you cannot unsee it. So, in order to correct this problem, we need to train the knee according to how it was built to move.

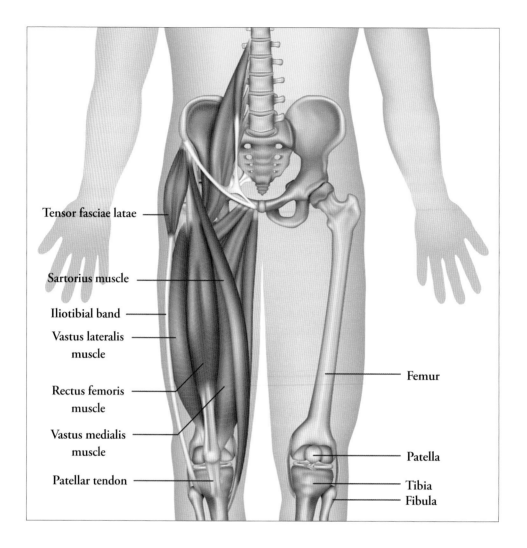

Tensor fasciae latae

Sartorius muscle

Iliotibial band

Vastus lateralis
muscle

Rectus femoris
muscle

Vastus medialis
muscle

Patellar tendon

Femur

Patella

Tibia
Fibula

2: Controlling Quad Function

Muscles contract and relax. Going from being in a relaxed state to a contracted state is one goal, but a more important skill is to be able to control going from a contracted state to a relaxed one. This is known as the *eccentric phase of movement* (see Calf Un-Raises on page 33 for an example of this). Concentric movement is used in gyms all over the world, but eccentric movement seems to be forgotten. You'll have an opportunity in the final two exercises of this chapter to find all the benefits of learning to eccentrically work your quads.

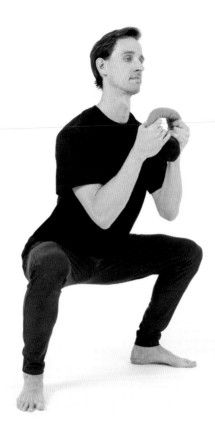

3: Progressive Loading Strategies

The best long-term solution for total knee health is to increase the volume of load you can sustain, or in other words, increase how much weight your knee can comfortably carry. Pain and injury occur when load exceeds your capacity. So, by increasing your capacity, you decrease your chances for pain and injury. You can't go wrong by getting strong. And you get strong by doing more than you did the day before. The best things aren't rushed.

An Important Note before Stretching

Before you go on to more complicated stretches or exercises for the knee, you need to make sure you have the appropriate joint spacing. Otherwise, you are doing stretches and exercises from an imbalanced base. It's not impossible to rehabilitate your knee without this joint space, but you will have to make concessions to maintain progress. In the stretches to come, we will work on joint spacing, then move to movements that target quad function and increasing your load.

THE STRETCHES

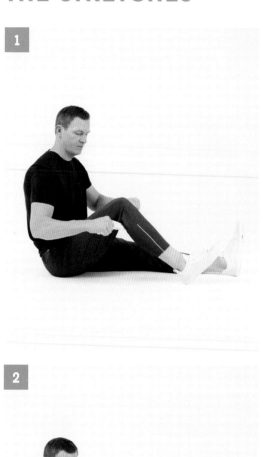

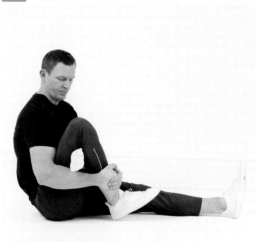

Towel Bends

This is perhaps the safest and easiest way to find relief for your knee pain. The towel tucked high up behind your knee provides leverage to gently create some space in your knee joint. Creating this space not only provides relief but prepares you for the stretches and exercises that follow.

Step 1: Place a rolled-up towel underneath the knee as closely behind the knee joint as possible. Pull your shin toward your body, flexing your knee.

Step 2: With the rolled-up towel under the knee you will begin to open the knee joint the more you pull the foot to the hip. Pulling and keeping the knee in this flexed position itself will begin to give space to the knee joint.

Step 3: You can use your hands to grab your shin and pull it closer to your body. If you push your shin back against your grip, it can help release more tension. Some people even find it helpful to do this in little bursts. If you begin to push the lower leg against the pressure of your hands without allowing any movement (*isometric contraction*), you can begin to release the tension in some of the muscles that are restricting full flexion.

Step 4: Holding the knee fully bent as you press against your hands 10 to 15 times should begin to create space in the knee. Upon releasing the position, slowly straighten and flex the knee to get the blood flow to return before standing up.

Two Helpful Variations

Here are two variations of this stretch. The directions follow the same logic, except you can do the position either lying down or kneeling if you find that more comfortable to start.

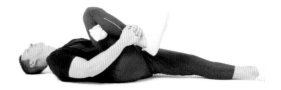

Note: By rolling up the towel to be thicker, you can create more space in the knee, but you will need to start by finding a comfortable thickness. You may notice this stretch more after you finish than while you are doing it, but keep your knee bent for at least 60 seconds even if you do not feel much happening in the stretch itself.

Most people find benefit in doing small contractions in their most flexed position. Keeping the flexed position and only allowing a few millimeters of movement seems to help open the joint space.

You will also notice more benefits if you maintain this flexed position between 90 seconds and 3 minutes.

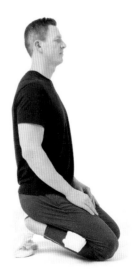

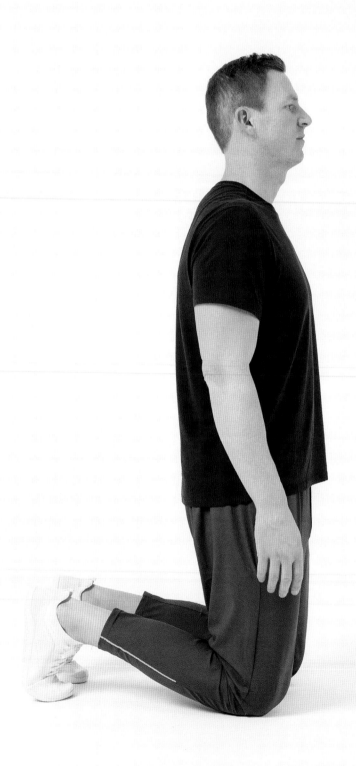

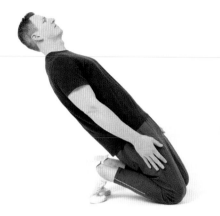

1B

Quad Control: Reverse Nordic Curls

Oftentimes exercises are only thought of in terms of creating an overpowering force, and that's important, but a vital component of your knee is your ability to absorb force. For your knee it's the quadricep muscles that are responsible for absorbing this force, and in this exercise you'll be learning how to do just that.

Step 1: Starting with both knees on the ground and your torso upright, slowly lean your chest back, going back as far as you can. The goal here is to lean back as far as you can, then return to the upright position. Most people begin by going back a few inches, but within a few days of practice you'll be able to go much farther.

Step 2: Return to the starting position.

Step 3: Repeat 3 to 5 times.

> **Note:** As you lean back, you'll begin to feel tension in the front of the thighs and abs. If you feel a pinch or pain in the low back, tuck the bottom of your pelvis forward like you are scooting forward in a chair. If you need further assistance completing the exercise correctly, try the band-assisted variation shown in the following stretch variations.

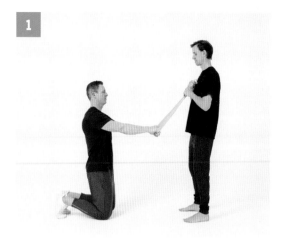

Second Variation

You can use a thick rubber band attached to a door hinge, pole or otherwise stable object, or a partner's hand, to help you lean back farther and also to help you return to the starting position. The goal is to train your quad muscles to learn to let go and to yield to the force of your lengthening. This can be jarring at first, but with a little bit of consistency you'll notice your body adapting.

Step 1: From the kneeling position, hold on to a thick rubber band as assistance for leaning backward and pulling yourself forward.

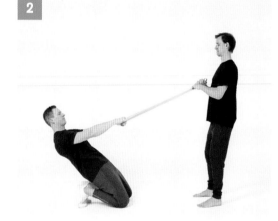

Step 2: Maintain an upright torso position, and keep your hips forward as you slowly move backward. Then use the band as much as you need to but as little as possible to return.

Helpful Variation: Tall Kneeling to Child's Pose Sitting

Learning to flex and extend the knee without the feet can be a very useful tool in learning how to load the knees. This is also in alignment with the idea that we need to train the knees to move forward and back with little to no rotation. The key here is to treat the movement as if it were a bridge by focusing your movement through the hips with the knees being a secondary factor.

Step 1: Keep the chest upright, and move from tall kneeling to sitting on the heels. This is a great way to free the hips and remove excessive strain on the knees.

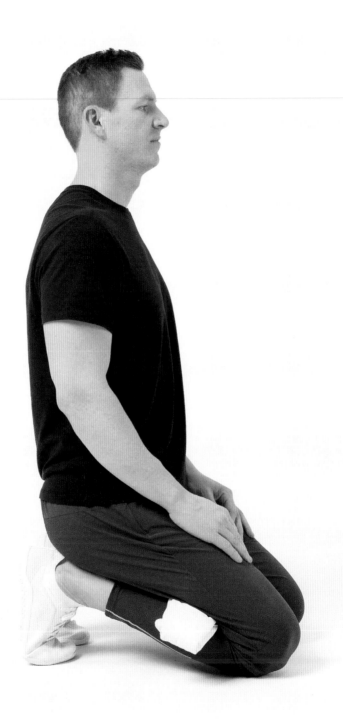

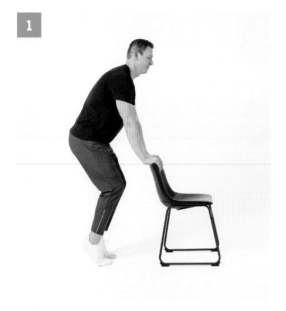

Heels-Up Squats

After opening up the joint space and learning to yield, it's time to put it all together. The Heels-Up Squat combines everything you have learned so far and adds a few new dimensions. The biggest thing this will do for your knees is not that it will teach you how to overpower and create force, but rather that it will allow you to build strong, resilient knees that are able to withstand all sorts of torque.

Step 1: Have all your weight on your forefoot: the ball of the foot just below the toes. You should take special care to keep the great toe and the ball of the foot down the entire time (as discussed in the foot and ankle chapter on page 25) to create a stable base. Do not lose your base! After you have created a stable base at the foot, you may notice you need balance assistance. Use a chair or wall to help you balance as much as you need but as little as possible. Most of the weight and pressure should be on the feet and legs.

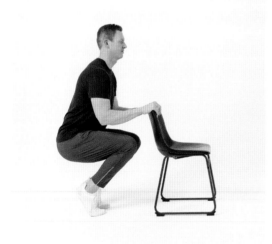

Step 2: Once you have these two points of stability, it's as simple as bending your knees as if you are sitting, then straightening them to propel yourself upright. Take care to go slowly, maintain your base of support and allow the bulk of the workload to be felt in the middle of your muscle (not the joints). Allow the knee to go over the toes or lean back into the hips to adjust where you sense the strain. The goal here is to adjust your body so that you are able to feel the pressure in the muscles above your knee and not in the knee joint.

Note: This exercise enforces proper form and demands you start slow. If you feel you are not able to do this movement without feeling strain in the knee joint and not the muscle, then you should revert to the Reverse Nordic Curl exercise (page 43) or really begin to focus on how you are keeping your weight on your feet. But once you are able to perform this movement correctly, then it's about trying to add more repetitions to create a strong and healthy knee. Initially, you should try to do 3 to 5 reps well. If you are able to get to 10 to 15, you will have the kind of knee that is going to be difficult to injure.

MOVING FORWARD

The knee bends and straightens with very little rotation. Over-rotating your knee causes torque. If you want a healthy knee, you need to be able to bend fully, move correctly and then add strength to keep the changes you have made.

"Perseverance is not a long race; it's many short races one after another."

—WALTER ELLIOT

"Character consists of what you do on the third and fourth tries."

—JAMES MICHENER

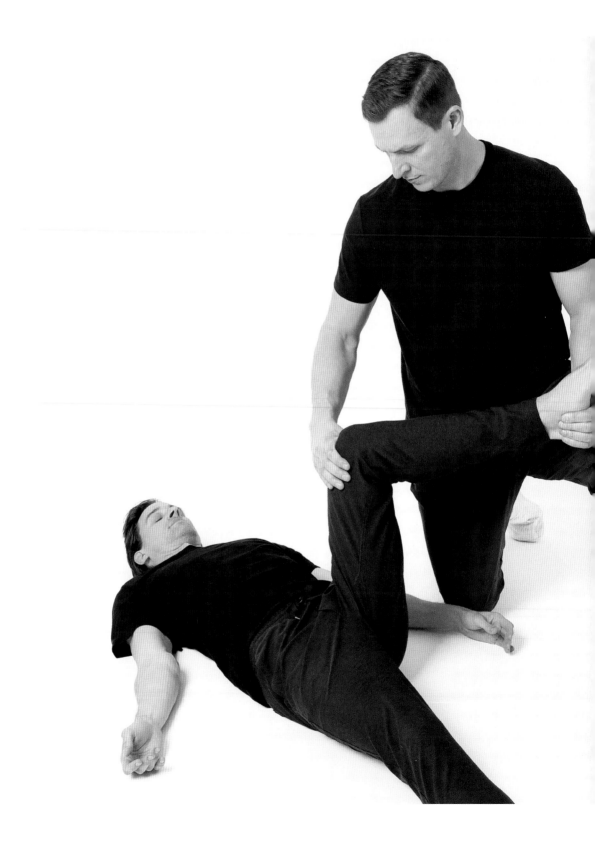

3D HIPS

How Internal Rotation Keeps Our Hips (and Low Back) Young

Spend some time with anyone scheduled for a hip replacement and you will instantly bear witness to the consequences of losing rotation. They will be unable to squat; they cannot twist or pivot; they will have, for the time being, given up golf or tennis; they shuffle or waddle when they walk and they are often in quite a lot of pain.

Rotation is the secret ingredient to speed and power and grace. From record-breaking home runs to gold-medal figure-skating performances, hip rotation in particular plays the crucial role of connecting the powerful lower body with the upper body via the pelvis and spine. Lose hip rotation and we sever the connection between our two halves and deny ourselves anything like our true athletic potential.

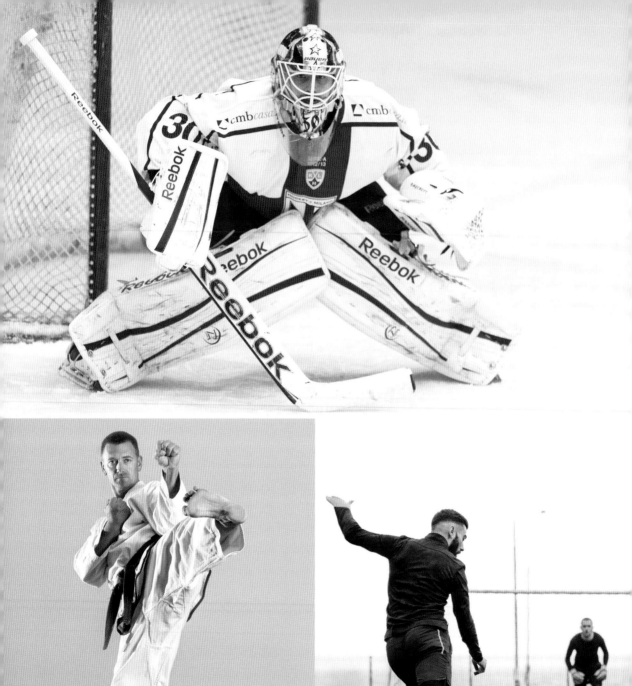
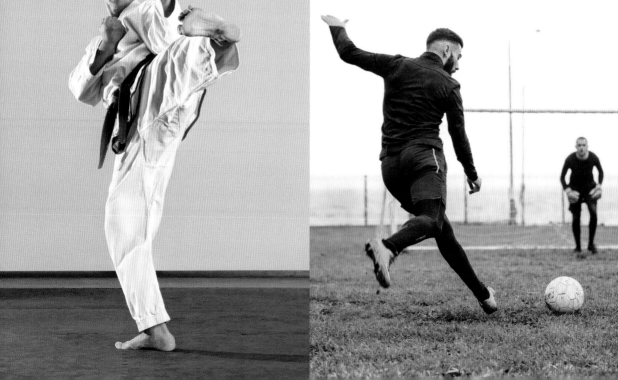

WHY THE HIPS NEED TO ROTATE

The hip, as opposed to a hinge joint (e.g., the knee), is a *ball and socket joint* (like the handles on a urinal or arcade joysticks). It may not be too far out of line to say that ball and socket joints, aside from our brains, are most responsible for *allowing* our bodies to move gracefully, with power and speed.

Human locomotion, in contrast to robots you'd see in older movies, is a constant display of three-dimensional movement. Even something that appears to be linear and two-dimensional, such as a squat, requires rotation of the hips, knees, ankles and pelvis. When rotation is lost, arthritic robotic movement is imminent, and toilet seats to rest on will be mandatory.

Thankfully, people do not, in fact, move like robots. We require rotation to accomplish any movement. For example, we must have at least 5 degrees of hip internal rotation just to walk without compensation (an alternative but less optimal strategy). We cannot safely squat deeply without adequate internal rotation of the hip. We couldn't pitch a baseball, hit a penalty kick in soccer or compete in martial arts, and we certainly would never make it to the NHL as a goalkeeper.

HOW A LOSS OF INTERNAL ROTATION CAN LEAD TO LOW BACK PAIN

What is much more common than hip pain? Low back pain. Yet, ironically, a common driver of low back pain is bad hips.

The hip complex comprises of the *head* (top) of the *femur* (upper leg bone) and the *acetabulum* (socket) of the *ilium (*pelvis). The spine integrates with the pelvis via the *sacrum* (the tailbone, the termination of the spine). Therefore, when the hip is locked and movement is restricted, you can now imagine that the femur bone in the photo is acting as a large wrench, and the hip socket behaves as the figurative bolt. That "wrench" now cranks on the entire pelvis as it moves. Bringing the leg up toward the chest will force the spine to bend forward. Bringing the leg behind the body will force the pelvis forward and slam the low back into an arched position. Bringing the leg out to the side of the body will force the hip to hike upward and the spine to bend toward the leg in a scoliotic fashion. All this leads to excessive shear, compression and friction within the spine. Once this happens, it's just a battle of survival: What will wear out first?

It is, therefore, imperative that we restore our hip internal rotation. Maybe you have no interest in being a goalkeeper, but we all want our spines to age well. We all want to pick up our kids, and our kids' kids.

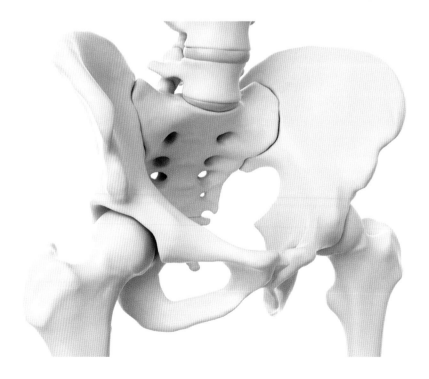

WHAT IS CAUSING YOUR HIP PAIN?

When crucial hip internal rotation is lost, things start to pinch and compress. The rim of the hip socket gets pinched, tissues get rubbed, sacroiliac joints get smashed and vertebrae shear across each other.

In the clinic I prefer to demonstrate to patients how nontraumatic injuries start to hurt over time. I flick them. Not hard in the head like my father used to do to me when I talked back as a child, but just a gentle finger flick against their forearm. "Does this hurt?" I ask. "No," they unanimously respond. I then say, "Just wait; it will. . . ."

Some don't believe me, and I keep flicking until they can't take it anymore and pull away. The truth is that such a gentle flick, which wouldn't hurt a toddler, eventually makes large bearded men whimper. How? A flick at a time. We call this *sensitization*. If you flick someone once, nothing happens. But as you keep doing it, it becomes red. Do it long enough and it will swell and become severely inflamed or blister. Continue to flick them even longer and you are likely to rupture the skin completely and force a bleed.

This is how that hip, when nothing happened at all, starts hurting one day. Small pinches and compressions, gentle shears and frictions over time. Accumulation.

Another analogy to help understand the tearing of a muscle or labrum is to imagine a knife on a rope. If you remember in *The Goonies* when they are trying to find all the hidden treasure of One-Eyed Willy, they set in motion a booby trap in which a blade slices across a rope that holds massive boulders. One slice does nothing, two the same, but eventually it goes, and with it a cascade of problems.

Remembering the End Goal

This may sound a tad obvious, but in order to restore hip rotation, we need to *rotate*. Ball and socket joints are metaphorical dogs, and rotation is their metaphorical stick. They are begging for it, and so delighted once they get it.

Be patient. Remember the idea of water and rocks when you are trying to improve the human body. A single day of water will not smooth the edges of a rock, but water *and time* will.

THE STRETCHES

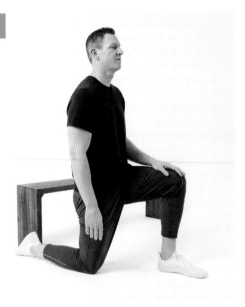

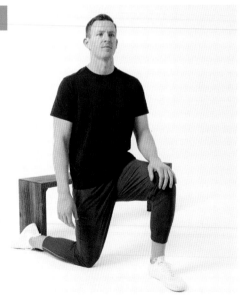

Half-Kneeling Internal Rotation

Here, we will begin training and acquiring greater internal rotation of the hip.

Step 1: In the half-kneeling position, rotate the back foot outward as far as comfortably possible (internal hip rotation), and block it with something immovable.

Step 2: Keeping an upright posture and your glutes contracted, gently rotate the torso toward the down leg until a medium stretch is felt.

Step 3: Hold this position for 60 to 90 seconds.

Step 4: Contract into the object for 10 seconds followed by relaxing for 10 seconds. Repeat this pattern for another 1 to 2 minutes.

Note: You can use a pillow under the down knee if kneeling is painful.

Hip Airplane

This stretch will train hip strength and hip control both into and out of internal rotation.

Step 1: Stand with one hand on a chair or wall for balance, with the opposite hand at your hip.

Step 2: Keeping the head-spine-leg in alignment, bend forward and lift the leg on the side of the body where the hand is at the hip.

Step 3: Stabilize and control this position at approximately 45 degrees.

Step 4: Focus all your effort on using the standing leg's hip muscles to control and move the body. Slowly rotate the body down over the standing leg until you can no longer rotate. Pause for 2 to 3 seconds.

Step 5: Squeeze the standing-leg glute to rotate the body away until you can no longer rotate. Be sure to only use the chair for balance, not to help you do the movement.

Step 6: Hold this position for 2 to 3 seconds. Repeat this stretch 5 to 10 times.

2

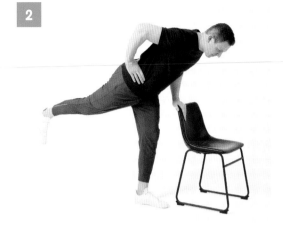

3

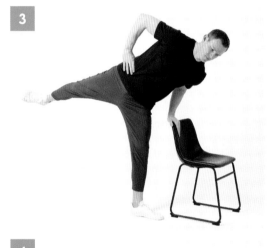

4

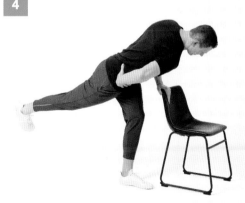

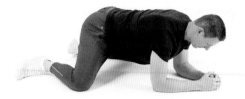

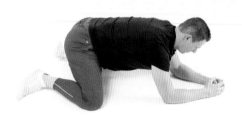

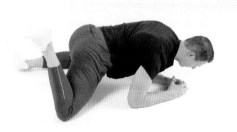

Tactical Frog

This movement's end goal is to actively recruit internal rotation. The first two movements are primarily passive, so now we will be using our muscles (with a little bit of momentum) to force rotation of the hip.

Step 1: Start by getting on your hands and knees. Slowly slide the knees apart until a stretch is felt with mild to no discomfort. The feet will be turned out so that the insides of the feet are against the floor. Try to keep the shins parallel with the spine.

Step 2: The Tactical Frog begins by rocking back toward your feet. Find a strong but comfortable stopping point.

Step 3: From there, we will keep our spine parallel to the floor and slide our body forward over our hands.

Step 4: At the end of this forward motion, we will take one leg at a time and attempt to rotate the leg off the ground as high as possible.

Step 5: Rock back toward the heels again and repeat but this time rotating and lifting the opposite foot.

Step 6: Repeat this movement in a dynamic rocking fashion, using some gentle momentum to help achieve hip internal rotation.

MOVING FORWARD

Losing hip rotation, most commonly internal rotation, will be the quickest way to ensure you progress to moving poorly and losing athleticism. Restoring and/or maintaining this internal rotation is fundamental to good-quality movement and maintaining the health of the hips and spine. As you gain small improvements in this ability, this will become evident by the way you are able to move, as well as the quality of comfort in and around the hips.

*"Do not go gentle
into that good night,*

*Old age should burn and
rave at close of day;*

*Rage, rage against
the dying of the light."*

–DYLAN THOMAS

*"Every avalanche begins with
the movement of a single snowflake . . .
[and] my goal is to move a snowflake."*

–THOMAS FREY

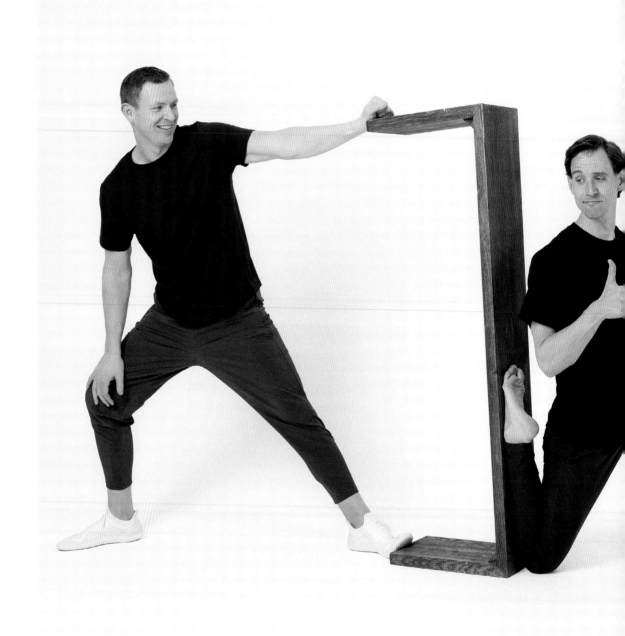

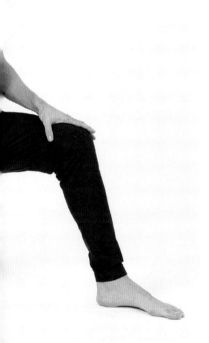

BOOTY-DRIVEN LIFE

How a Strong and Flexible Foundation Relieves Low Back Pain

Strengthening your glutes will relieve your back pain, but sitting can cause the opposite to happen. Sitting allows your hips to bend in the front. This is called hip flexion. The opposite of flexion is extension. The idea is that because your hips are flexed so often, the opposing motion (hip extension) becomes lacking; therefore, to make up for this lack of hip extension, you overuse (overextend) your spine and back muscles, which leads to pain. But if you did have full hip extension, of which strong glutes are a sign, your back would feel much less stress because the hips are able to finally do their job. Restoring hip extension allows you to use your glutes; you'll have a life driven by your booty and not your low back.

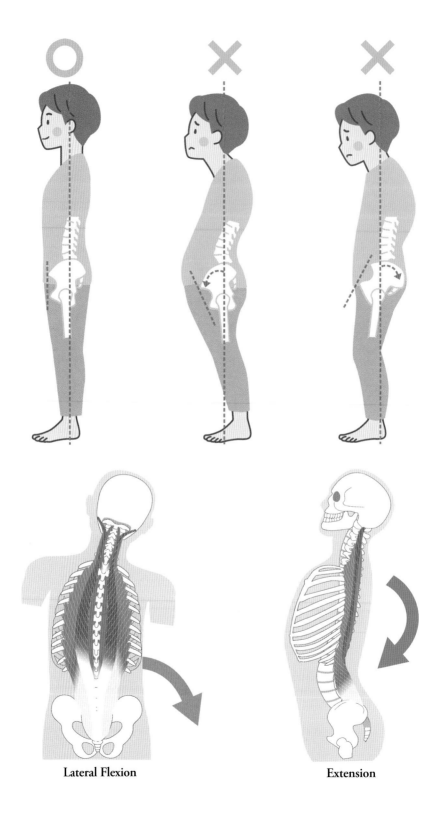

Lateral Flexion

Extension

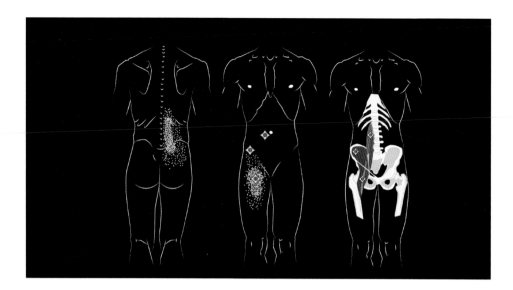

WHAT IS CAUSING YOUR PROBLEM?

By repetitively using the smaller joints and muscles of the low back without also engaging in hip extension (this is where the glutes are working), you overstrain smaller structures instead of spreading the workload out evenly. Your hips have so well accommodated to the bent position of sitting that the opposite range of motion (hip extension) has become limited, and now you might be using your spine to make up for this lack of hip extension.

This is the slow drip of aches that, over time, build up until one sneeze freezes you in bed for a few days. This type of back pain is usually not bad most of the time, but you know it's there. You are able to do most things, or you may have found new ways to do things to avoid triggering the pain. You may know exactly how far you can walk or how long you can sit. This is not like a broken bone from a fall. This is the slow accumulation of unhelpful habits.

WHY YOUR BACK ISN'T GETTING BETTER

As your low back becomes tense, it would seem to make sense that stretching the muscles of the low back would help, but this approach fails for two reasons:

1. The "dose" of your stretch does not match the intensity of your problem.

2. It fails to address the root cause.

As described earlier, if your problem has been slowly building over time, it will be hard to get the teeter-totter of health to swing in your direction with just a few simple low back stretches. This approach will work if you are addressing the primary problem and your efforts exceed the intensity of your problem. This is a tough combination that many find challenging.

You need to outstretch your problem.

Tips on Finding the Right Stretch

The right balance can be hard to strike. Either the stretch is too easy, too boring and doesn't do anything or it's too hard and you just don't want to do it again. The proper balance is right at the upper limit of your capabilities. You can do it, but it's not comfortable. Finding this dosage often engages what science calls the *flow state:* a well-researched mental and physical state in which you are challenged but you can meet this challenge. Learning and progress tend to happen easily when you discover how to strike that balance.

The first of the stretches in this chapter is known as a Hip Flexor Stretch (page 64). If done correctly, it can begin to correct many of the problems listed in this chapter. After that, we will show you progressively more challenging stretches that accomplish the same goal of training the hip to pull its weight. You want to find the stretch that helps you sense your hip is moving without stressing your low back (the root cause) while also finding one that challenges you enough to cause your body to adapt (proper dosage). These exercises all address the same cause, but you will be responsible for finding which one benefits you the most. Once you find your match, it's simply about doing it so much that it becomes easy.

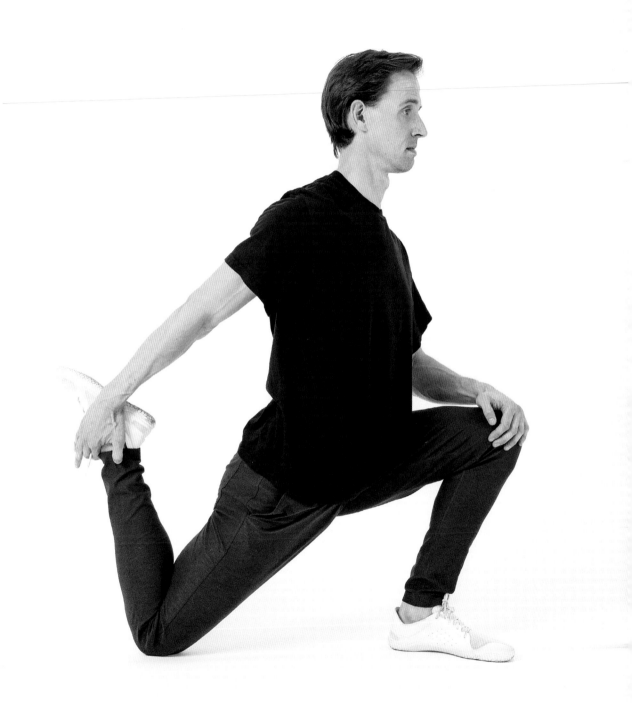

THE STRETCHES

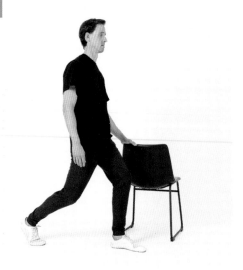

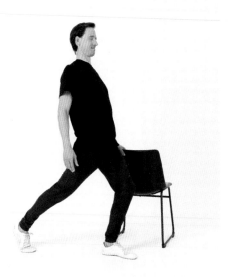

The Hip Flexor Stretch

First, establish the correct position. Second, move into the stretch. Third, focus on how long you can hold the stretch, also called "time under tension." Establishing proper position allows us to target the intended muscular area and maximize our time under tension. The more time under tension we can manage, the more change we can make.

Step 1: Standing, exhale the ribs down, and tilt the bottom of the pelvis forward.

Step 2: Take one step forward, and shift your weight onto the front foot, then push off the back. Be sure to keep the bottom of the pelvis forward as you lean onto the front leg.

Step 3: Feel a stretch in the front of the thigh on the back leg; breathe 5 times or hold for 90 seconds. Do not lose your pelvic or spinal position.

Note: You are looking to feel a stretch on the front of the thigh that is close to but not exceeding your limits of discomfort while not arching your low back. Your low back should be straight. If you notice this has become easy for you to do, it means your body is beginning to adapt. Many will feel relief here and stop, but if you're looking for lasting results, it's vital you try to make more progress.

Variation 1: Challenge Yourself

People practice this stretch for years and still discover ways in which it opens up the body. I have been doing it for over a decade now, and it always reveals space where I can improve, whether it's that I can make the stretch deeper or control my breathing (slow and low). Or perhaps it's that I can hold the position for a longer period of time, bend the knee forward or the back leg farther back or move with my torso more upright. There are books written on the topic of this stretch. It's unfortunate that it only gets a page here, but I do hope you spend some time with this one. It's got a lot to give if you're willing to take the time.

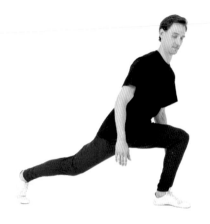

Step 1: Repeat steps 1 through 3 from the previous exercise, but take a larger step.

Step 2: Bend the knees a bit more to increase the tension.

Step 3: Increase the amount of time and tension to new limits.

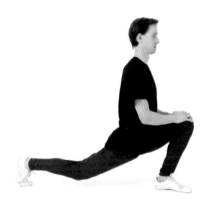

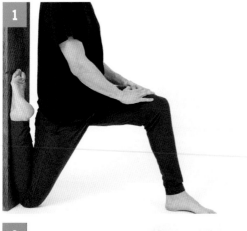

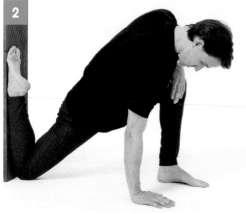

The Couch Stretch

Deceptively named, the couch stretch has very little to do with comfort and everything to do with hip extension. Putting the foot against a couch (or bed or wall) flexes the knee and further isolates the position of hip extension. If I were trapped on a desert island and could only do one stretch ever again, I would choose this stretch. With a minimal amount of consistency, this stretch will prove beneficial. It is scalable to almost every decade of life. It can be made very simple and accessible but can quickly become challenging. Whether you're looking to unwind from sitting all day or warming up for a CrossFit workout, there is some level of this stretch for you.

Step 1: Place your flexed knee in the corner of your couch so that your shin and thigh are as vertical as possible. Keep your upper bodyweight on the front leg as you shift forward onto the front leg.

Step 2: Tuck the bottom of your pelvis forward as you lean on the front leg. You should feel a stretch in the front of the thigh.

Step 3: Keep the torso forward over the knee until you feel a good stretch in the front of the hip. Once you notice the hip stretch, you can begin to raise the torso up. Hold the stretch: For easy, go for 60 seconds. For average, go for 2 minutes. For excellent, attempt 5 minutes.

Note: The key again here is the sequence. Except it's a completely new sequence. Starting from position 1, you may not notice much of a stretch, but you have naturally stacked your femur, pelvis and spine in your neutral position. You no longer need to focus on your core position as we begin. It has already been set for you. Pinning the knee back and the opposite leg forward (position 1) with your torso forward means we have trapped the irrelevant movements. The only movement left wide open is hip extension. The more you shift forward, the more you must extend the down knee.

Helpful Variation: Ground or Chair Assistance

You can do this movement on the ground or using a couch with a chair in front of you for support. If it helps you maintain the tension in the front of the thigh without extending your back, any type of assistance is welcomed.

MOVING FORWARD

In this chapter we covered how the problem of hip extension due to sitting for too long can lead to overactivity and irritation of the low back. So, by replacing excessive low back extension with hip extension, we begin to reverse the problem.

The final consideration is the amount of time it will take until you notice a difference. For some it will be a few days, whereas for others it may take weeks, but with a minimum amount of consistency you'll get there.

"Everything is walking distance if you have the time."

−STEVEN WRIGHT

"Without long practice one cannot suddenly understand. . . ."

−TAI CHI PROVERB

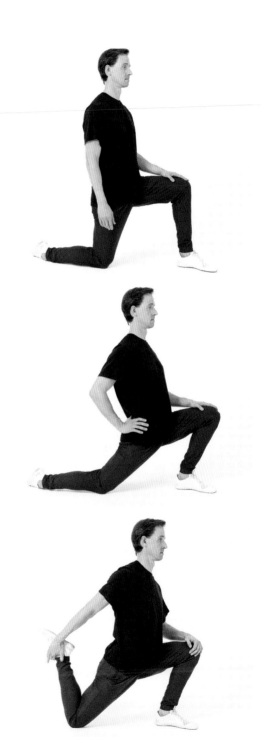

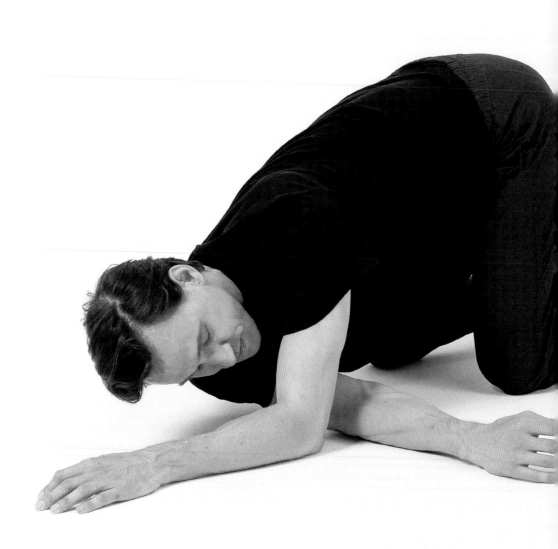

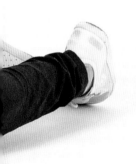

THORACIC ROTATION

How Trunk Rotation Restores Athleticism

The most basic principle of movement is that a thing can move because it is propelled off of a stable base, like pushing a boat from a secure dock. The lower body moves from the ground, but the "ground" for the upper body is the core.

Your core is not your abdominal muscles. Your core is the internal pressure of your abdomen that extends from the upper dome of your diaphragm to the lower bowl of the pelvic floor. This egg-shaped pressure system is mostly controlled by another pressure system encaged by your ribs and wrapped around your heart: your lungs.

Learning to gain control over this ground is fundamental to proper movement of the upper body. The muscles in your neck, shoulders and upper back may be tight to make up for the lack of control over your internal tension. But learning to create and control this inner tension often helps relieve the chronic external tightness, which is exactly what we are going to work on in this chapter.

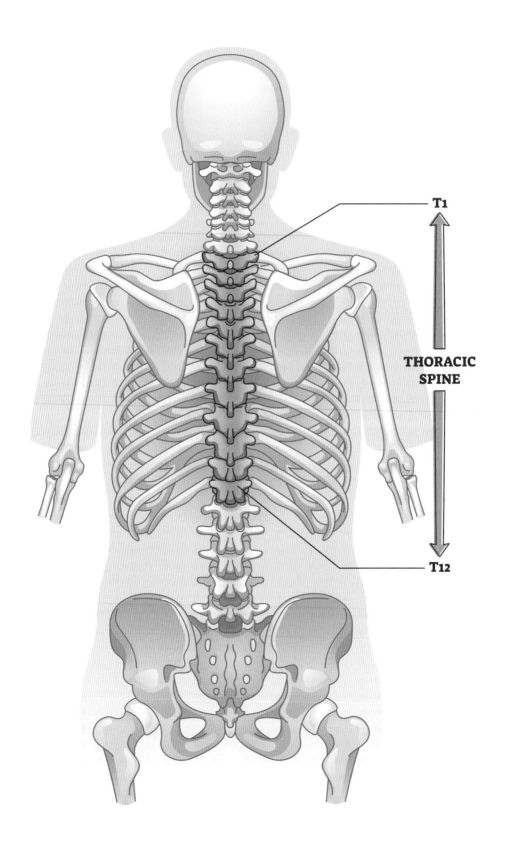

T1

THORACIC
SPINE

T12

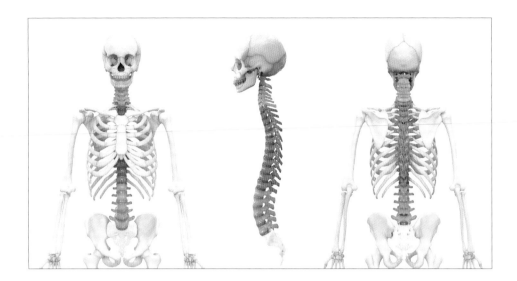

WHY TRUNK ROTATION MATTERS

All movement is rotational movement. Your body is not a linear system. The biggest area of rotation and the biggest *center* of rotation are in your trunk. It rotates, but everything else rotates around it. So, if the internal foundation is imbalanced, the external muscular system will create tension to maintain normality.

The neck and the upper back muscles are the common victims of core imbalances. The neck muscles having to work to lift the rib cage upward almost cancels their ability to help you rotate your neck if left unaddressed. The muscles in the mid- and upper back are also often required to stay in a contracted, spasmed state because of the lack of internal pressure in the back of your core.

Having proper trunk rotation evenly to the left and right is one of the first signs your core is in a balanced state. Increasing your ability to rotate is the easiest way to realize and then clear out these imbalances.

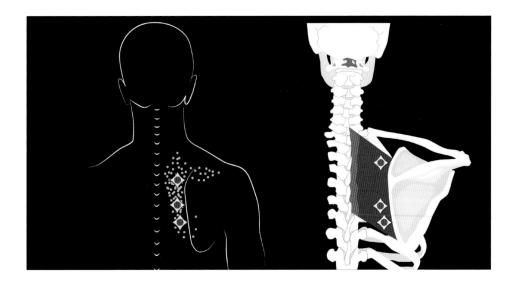

WHAT'S ACTUALLY HAPPENING HERE?

When you feel pain in the torso, typically between or below the shoulder blades in the back, people are often unaware of how that pain began. There is rarely a dramatic incident connected to the pain here; instead, the pain is described as involuntarily showing up one day. But this pain comes with a few clues that might help us solve this mysterious problem.

You may feel the limitations of the stiffness in your movement, or you may notice triggers or areas of pain that people refer to as knots. This pain has a purpose, and the more clearly you understand why you have this, the easier it will be to unwind the problem.

This pain secretly steals movement. When your movement becomes limited, so does your strength. This process happens so slowly it is hardly noticeable until it's too late. But in reversing the process, you may also gain movement and strength before the pain fully resolves.

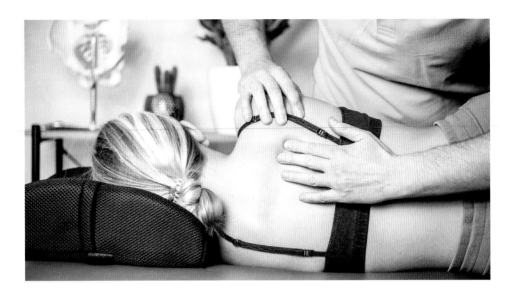

WHAT IS THE DEEPER PROBLEM?

At the most extreme points of pain in this area, you may find taking a deep breath to be sharp and painful. This is a major clue as to the nature of the problem. The secret movement of the rib cage and torso is your breathing. Yes, there is rotation and counterrotation, but breathing is the key to controlling the internal pressure, which leads to controlling the external tension as well.

This is why most of the problems here are hard to explain. Breathing involuntarily into poor postures strains the natural expansion and compression that should take place, until your body requires an unnatural compensation to maintain itself. It's a very subtle, slow, sneaky process.

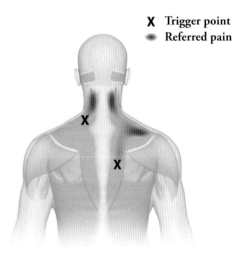

X Trigger point
● Referred pain

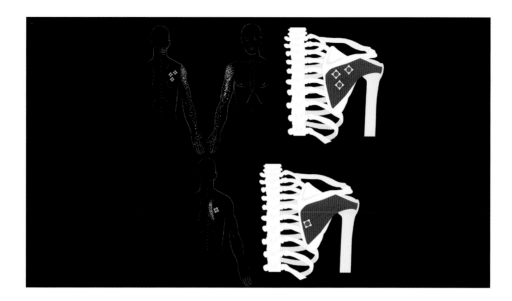

There is a theory that we adopt a posture only because it is easy to breathe in that posture. It's comfortable in that position. Getting out of that position is usually where you notice the disturbance. While these postures make it easy to breathe in, they may not be beneficial for your muscles or joints to function as they should.

Your body sacrifices position and muscle tension to make breathing easy. So, if you want a better position and better muscle tension, you need to learn to control your breathing.

How Do We Control Our Breathing?

Breathing has two phases: inhalation and exhalation. And there are a set of muscles that help with each one. Generally, people have stronger inhalation muscles and weaker muscles of exhalation. So, the simplest way to begin to correct issues in the torso, ribs and core is simply to strengthen your muscles of exhalation by blowing up a balloon.

Strengthening the muscles of exhalation by blowing up a balloon is by far the simplest solution to 80 percent of the problems here. Encouraging exhalation is the body's natural muscle relaxer.

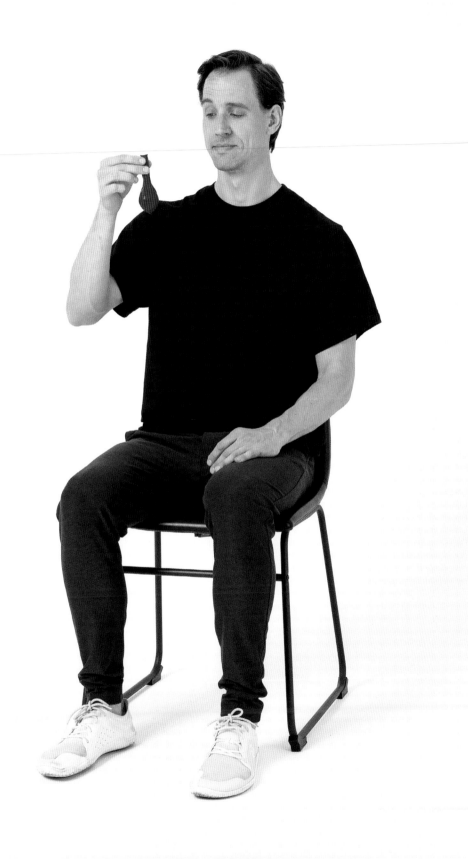

THE STRETCHES

Using a Balloon to Relax

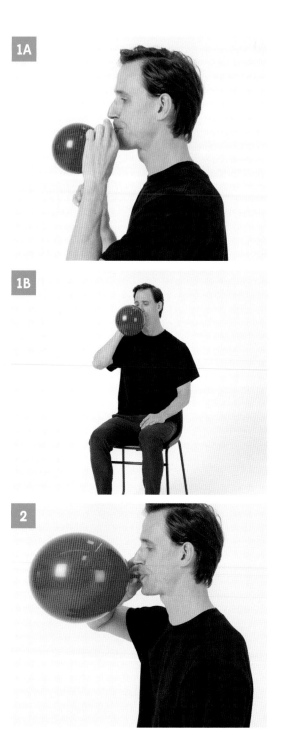

The most basic element of breathing is inhaling and exhaling. You want to be able to fully inhale and fully exhale. By pushing the limit of the spectrums on both ends, you are building a better neutral zone, or resting area for breathing. You don't want to be over-inhaling or under-exhaling. Instead, you want to create a nice big buffer zone between these two extremes. This drill will help develop a more natural, even breathing state.

Step 1: Breathe in through the nose and out into the balloon without allowing your cheeks to puff out. Rather, purse your lips as you blow up the balloon.

Step 2: Focusing on the exhale, breathe slowly in through your nose and out into the balloon until the balloon is full.

Step 3: Repeat 3 to 5 times. Being able to relax and easily blow up the balloon is the goal. You may notice you over-engage certain areas at first, but as you progress, you should be able to not strain while blowing up the balloon.

Thread the Needle

1

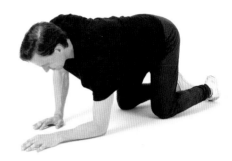

As you begin to correct breathing imbalances with the balloon, you'll also need to start to address the rotational asymmetries within the torso. Rotation is guided by reaching, but we also want to isolate movement to the torso, so we will use the child's pose position as we begin to train our rotation as well as breathing.

Step 1: From a kneeling position, place both elbows on the ground in front of the knees.

Step 2: Reach the right arm between the left elbow and left knee as far as you can, setting the back of the right shoulder on the ground.

Step 3: Breathe in this position.

Step 4: Once breathing has become comfortable, reach the left arm up to the sky. Again, breathe in this position at least 5 times, focusing on the exhale.

2

Step 5: Repeat on the opposite side.

Note: Your goal is to make both sides feel about the same. Once you can comfortably reach as far left as you can right, you have mastered this movement. Another sign you have mastered this movement is that you can comfortably breathe in either position.

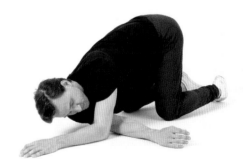

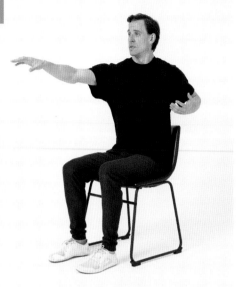

Seated Reaching Recipe

This final exercise is a recipe of the previous two exercises with a few new ingredients to help bring everything together. You already have breathing and rotation down, but now you'll be combining and synchronizing this with reaching. Because pain is isolating and breaks connections, beginning to use everything together is the ultimate goal.

Connecting reaching with breathing and rotation will help you learn to use all the pieces involved as one unit. Going fast or doing more reps here is not the goal. Rushing this movement will ruin the results.

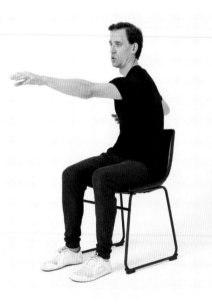

2

Before starting this exercise, there is an important note on your head position: Keep the head straight. Or keep your gaze fixed, and do not allow the rotation below the neck to pull or strain in the neck. If you notice your neck straining, you are rotating too far. Adjust your head position as needed to avoid straining the neck. You will notice huge shifts in your posture if you can master this exercise.

Step 1: Seated, simultaneously reach your right arm forward as you pull the left back. Inhale.

Step 2: Then exhale as you reach the left arm forward and pull the right arm back.

Step 3: Repeat this pattern 10 times, then reverse the pattern for the opposite side.

Step 4: Make sure to keep your head straight as everything else rotates.

MOVING FORWARD

Developing the ability to change direction by creating a stable core through your breathing and rib cage position is not simple. But if you can dedicate some of your time and attention to working on this just a little, you will notice profound changes in your movement and athleticism.

*"Change the way you
look at things, and the
things you look at change."*

–DR. WAYNE DYER

*"Those who cannot
change their minds
cannot change anything."*

–GEORGE BERNARD SHAW

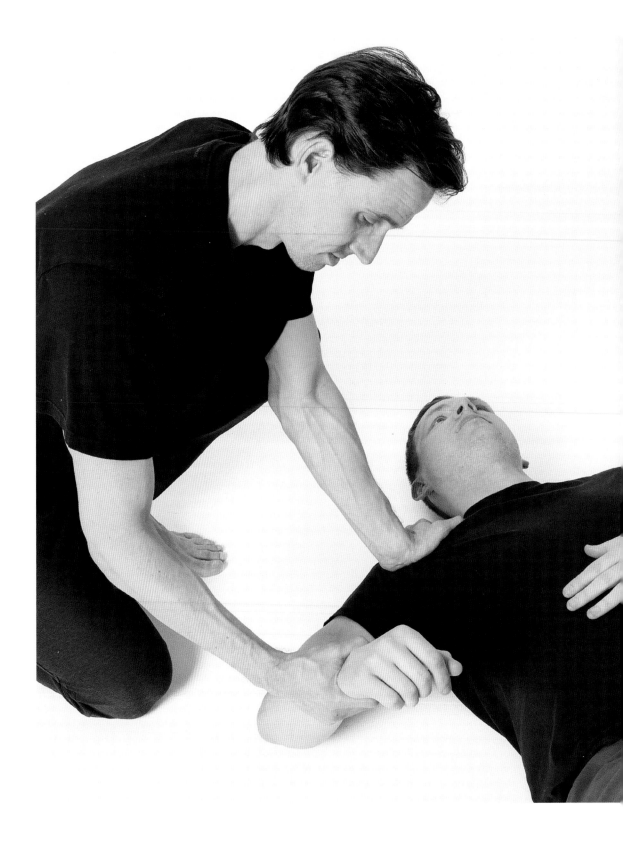

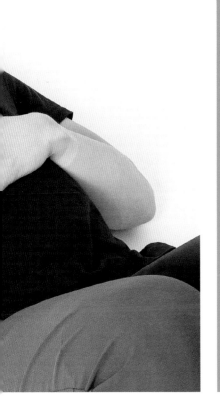

MONKEY SHOULDERS

How to Fix and Bulletproof Your Shoulders

Whenever I read any comic book or watch any film involving Spider-Man, one question that really irks me is: "Hey! How can Spider-Man's tiny toddler shoulders handle the massive trauma that would result from a one-armed overhead spiderweb swing from one skyscraper to the next?"

The stories go on to explain and even show the processes by which Spider-Man gains his knowledge and skills. But they never showcase his shoulder routine for us. Only a person—even a superhero, I propose—with an intricately well-developed and robust shoulder-movement routine, could withstand such a demanding vocation. Until such a routine is presented, I await the more realistic scene wherein the spiderweb swings his severed arm across Times Square.

The shoulder complex (glenohumeral joint) is the most mobile joint in the human body . . . and with that exceptional ability comes, yes, you guessed it, great responsibility. Let's take a look at why shoulder pain manifests and what we can do to correct it.

WHY DOES YOUR SHOULDER HURT?

Unless you are a superhero, we can assume that at some point in your life, you will likely come face-to-face with some troubling shoulder problems. The question is: Why?

When one peruses the research that has been conducted over the last hundred years, one can start to lay claims to the risks associated with developing shoulder pain. These risk factors include age, obesity, smoking, diabetes, emotional distress and occupation/ lifestyle. Within the category of occupation/lifestyle, we observe that heavy physical work and overhead, vibratory and repetitive actions, along with awkward postures, are risk factors for developing shoulder pain.

While such studies are important and should be considered, they fail to address what is (in our opinion) the most necessary and controllable risk factor: **disuse**. The classic adage "If you don't use it, you lose it" is more of a fact when it comes to biological tissue. The trade-off with the shoulder being the most mobile joint in our body is that it commensurately requires a vast range of capacity in order to maintain its health. When we regularly use our body in a dynamic capacity, we elicit adaptations within it. The fancy textbook term for this is *mechanotransduction*.

Mechanotransduction, in simplest terms, is the process by which physical or mechanical stress to human tissue gets translated into chemical signals that tell the body it needs to adapt. Start playing the guitar? Just wait a couple weeks, and your fingers will be calloused and no longer in pain. Want denser bones and larger muscles? Lift heavy weights.

Outsourced Shoulders

The fortunate, or rather unfortunate, reality of modern human living is that we have essentially outsourced our shoulder labor. We don't need to climb things, throw things or carry things to survive. Our shoulders can live out their cushy lives resting on couch arms, hanging flaccid on motor-propelled lawn mowers and with lackadaisical ease assisting the hand in picking up the telephone to call an arborist who can cut down all those overgrown trees for you. And yet, 18 million Americans alone each year are clinically affected by shoulder pain.

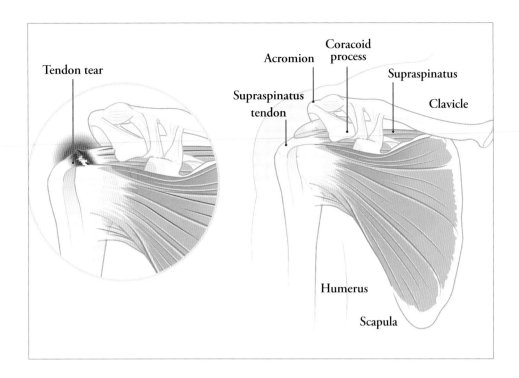

WHAT ARE THE PRIMARY CAUSES OF SHOULDER PAIN?

The four primary shoulder afflictions are rotator cuff injury, adhesive capsulitis (frozen shoulder), dislocations and osteoarthritis, with rotator cuff issues comprising the bulk of the complaints.

While it is helpful to understand which conditions are most common among the population, what matters most is why. We will not be addressing that in any major capacity (there are entire books written about the shoulder or just parts of it). But we will try to elucidate some major causes in the stretches to come.

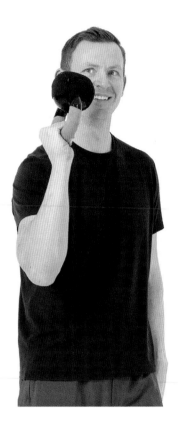

HOW TO UTILIZE MECHANOTRANSDUCTION TO BULLETPROOF THE SHOULDERS

In order to achieve the full range of motion involved in a healthy shoulder complex, we need to incorporate two primary objectives in the movement routine: rotation and load. The only way a shoulder joint achieves full pain-free movement is if the joint has the capacity to roll, spin and glide. This ability allows the hand and arm to move in a maximal three-dimensional capacity. Then we add load. The law of mechanotransduction tells us this load will trigger a sequence of events that will lay down new connective tissue making the components of the shoulder complex more robust, powerful and resilient. This law is not unique to the shoulder. Once this concept takes full shape in your mind, you will be able to use it to better understand how to rehab any future soft-tissue injury.

We have condensed the truly unlimited ways you can train the shoulders into a concise routine that has great potential to recover some of the youthful shoulder strength you once had.

THE STRETCHES

The Four-Way Stretch

1: Anterior Shoulder Capsule (ASC)

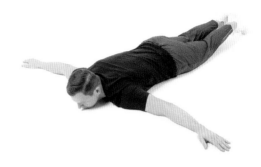

The goal of this stretch is to, over time, release any overt tension in the front of the shoulder and pectoral muscles to allow for better shoulder range of motion.

Step 1: Lie flat on your belly with your arms out like a T, or like Rose on the *Titanic*.

Step 2: Bring one arm into the push-up position.

Step 3: Using the hand in the push-up position, lift that side of the body, and roll it over and onto the opposite arm (the arm being stretched).

Step 4: Hold the stretch for at least 90 seconds.

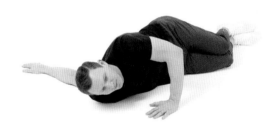

Step 5: Repeat on the other side.

> **Note:** It may not be exactly a T position. If any particular position is uncomfortable, then try going up or down a few degrees until the position feels like a stretch in the front of the shoulder *without* any pain.

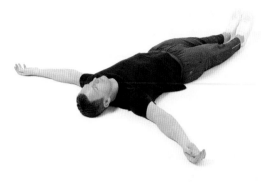

1

2: Posterior Shoulder Capsule (PSC)

The goal of this stretch is to, over time, release any overt tension in the back of the shoulder, therefore allowing more freedom of movement.

Step 1: Lie on your back in the *Titanic* position.

Step 2: Roll your body over and on top of the down arm (the arm you rolled toward).

Step 3: Place the free arm into the push-up position to control the load placed on the down (stretched) arm.

Step 4: Find a pain-free stretch, and hold it for at least 90 seconds.

Step 5: Repeat on the other side.

3

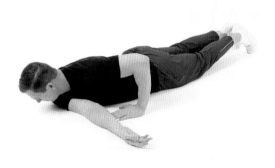

3: External Rotation (ER)

This movement will help you acquire passive external rotation over time.

Step 1: Stand facing a wall with your arm at your side, bend your elbow to 90 degrees and place your palm flat on the wall.

Step 2: Dig the elbow of that arm into the front of your hip bone to anchor it. Additionally add stability by placing the opposite arm on your bicep.

Step 3: Rotate your body away from the hand on the wall until you feel a deep stretch but no pain.

Step 4: Hold the stretch for at least 90 seconds.

Step 5: Repeat on the other side.

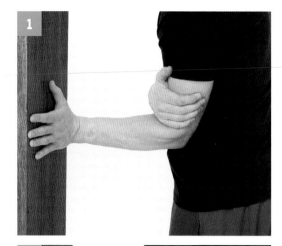

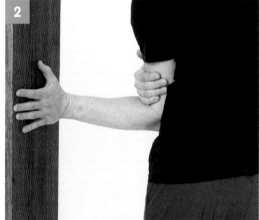

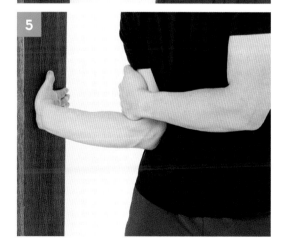

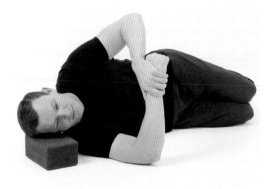

4: Internal Rotation (IR)

This movement will help you acquire passive internal rotation over time.

Step 1: Lying on your back with your arms in the T position, roll onto one side and bend your elbow to 90 degrees, with your palms facing your feet. You can use a block or pillow here to support your head and neck.

Step 2: Using your top hand, gently guide the bottom hand toward the floor until you feel a medium stretch. Be sure you do not have any sharp, pinching pain here.

Step 3: Hold this position for 90 seconds or more.

Step 4: Repeat on the other side.

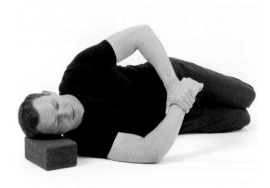

Loaded Internal Rotation

This stretch will help you build resilience within the rotator cuff by loading the internal rotators. Remember how this is essential to bulletproofing your shoulders. First we work on rotation, then we add load.

Step 1: Lying on your back with your arms in the T position, roll onto one side and bend your elbow to 90 degrees. With your palms facing your feet, hold a weighted household item (dumbbell, soup can, heavy hammer, etc.) in that same hand. You can use a block or pillow here to support your head and neck.

Step 2: Allow the weight to slowly, and without any jerking movement, fall toward the floor over a count of 8 to 10 seconds.

Step 3: Once you hit the end of your maximal safe range of motion, hold for another 5 seconds.

Step 4: Use your opposite free hand to assist the weight back to the starting position.

Step 5: Repeat 5 times.

Step 6: Repeat on the opposite side.

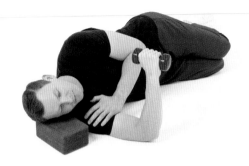

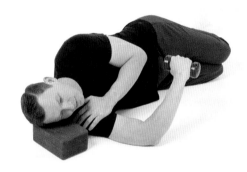

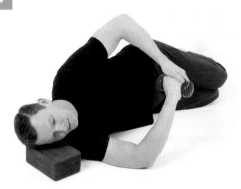

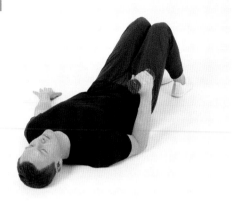

Loaded External Rotation

Here we will load the internal rotators and build resilience within the rotator cuff.

Step 1: Lying on your back in the now-famous T position, slide your elbow along the floor until it is against the side of your body, then bend the elbow 90 degrees, with your palm facing your belly.

Step 2: With a light weight in hand, begin to slowly, and with control, allow the weight to fall outward toward the floor over a period of about 8 to 10 seconds.

Step 3: After reaching your maximum safe rotation, hold for an additional 5 seconds.

Step 4: In this move you can choose to come back up with or without the help of the opposite hand.

Step 5: Repeat 5 times.

Step 6: Repeat on the opposite side.

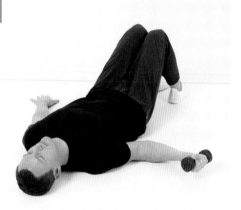

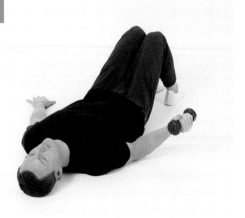

MOVING FORWARD

To paraphrase a famous saying, "The person who does not read has no advantage over the person who cannot read." The shoulder joint, with its extremely unique mobility and maneuverability, is a defining characteristic of human potential. However, many will never make any use of such abilities, relegating the shoulder joint to the banal tasks of simply reaching and shrugging.

If you have ever been to SeaWorld or witnessed a killer whale (orca) in captivity, you will notice the ubiquity of flopped-over dorsal fins. In the wild, these whales cruise through deep waters for miles and miles a day, constantly stressing the collagen fibers of their fins, keeping them flexible but strong and *upright*. It is typically only when these whales are not in their natural environment that disuse becomes obvious. As they spend most of their time at the surface of their tanks with much fewer miles traversed per day, the fins can no longer hold on to their original function.

The upside is that we do not need to be an Olympic gymnast or swim for miles every day to keep our shoulders healthy. Just a few minutes of full range of motion each day can be all we need to slow most age-related issues of the shoulder.

"And a lean, silent figure slowly fades into the gathering darkness, aware at last that in this world, with great power there must also come—great responsibility!"

—AMAZING FANTASY #15 (SPIDER-MAN)

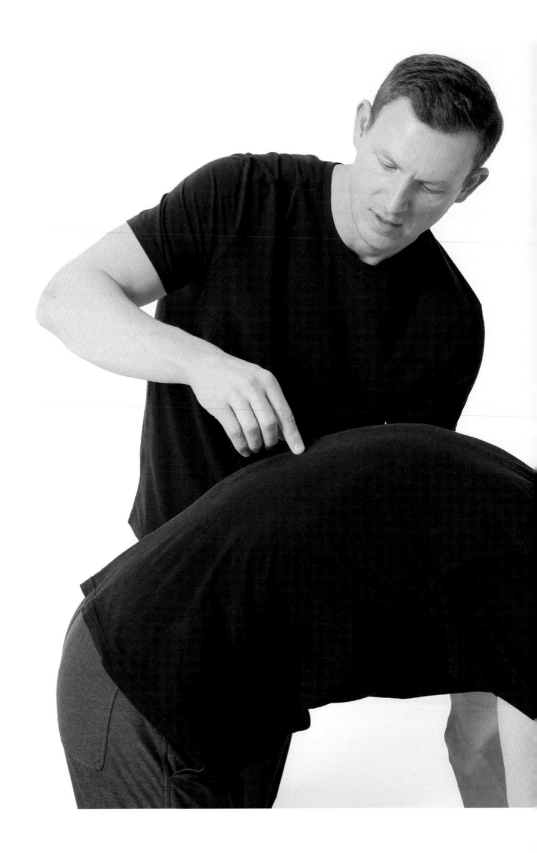

SALAMANDER SPINE

Why a Healthy Spine Means a Healthy Life

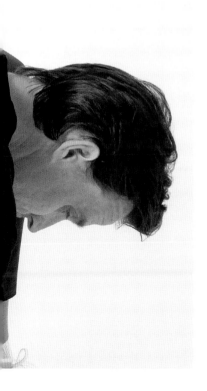

Bipedalism, having or using only two feet for locomotion, played a massive role in how humans evolved to acquire the mobile and robust shoulder abilities outlined in the previous chapter. By standing upright on only two limbs, we effectively unleashed our arms and hands to become amazingly adept tools. This unique trait comes to have an enormous impact on our spines. While bipedalism has a freeing effect on the shoulder, it seems to have been a burdensome evolutionary progression for the low back. Some studies have demonstrated that low back pain alone can be costlier to our health than all other musculo-skeletal conditions combined.

Walking on two legs isn't all bad. Energetically, this has allowed for an efficiency of movement that can hardly be matched. It allows for such dynamic interactions between the upper and lower body that it gives way to Olympic gymnastics and Cirque du Soleil®. With one small prerequisite: that we keep our spine healthy.

The dictionary defines spineless as "lacking strength of character." Not an adjective anyone wishes to be associated with. For the purposes of this book, spine-lessness will inevitably be synonymous with lacking a foundation. Lacking our one and only linchpin.

THE LINCHPIN OF THE BODY

In the days of the Oregon Trail and the centuries preceding Henry Ford, wagons were the primary mode of transport for cargo, goods and people. Among all the gadgetry, ropes, horses and planks of wood is a tiny invaluable item called a linchpin. A boring, simple item without which the entire wagon complex would be rendered useless.

This irreplaceable object fits into just the right place. An ingenious piece of metal so uncomplicated it reminds one of a toothpick or a fig leaf in a painting of a nude. What does it do? It keeps the wheels on the wagon.

Today, we use the word *linchpin* to portray something indispensable. "I don't know what I would do without my assistant; she is my linchpin." "We can't lay off Tom; he is the linchpin for the entire department."

Just as the linchpin to a well-made book is the health of its spine, the undisputed linchpin of human structure and function is also the spine.

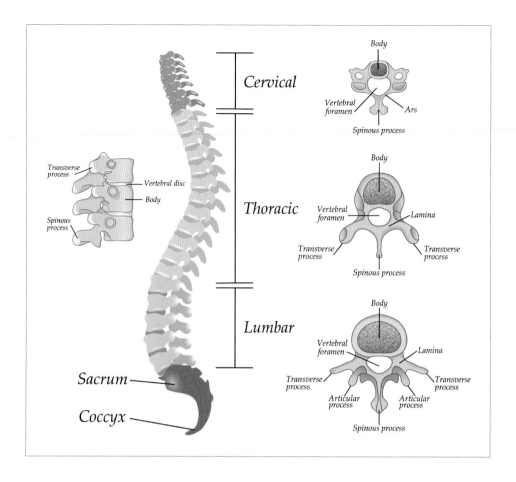

WHY DO WE HAVE SUCH BAD BACKS?

The first thing to understand about the human spine, in contrast to the linchpin, is that it is very complex. On paper the spine is simply 24 individual bones (typically) from three distinct regions of opposing curvature. 7 from the neck, 12 from the middle back and 5 in the lower spine that terminate on a fused sacrum and coccyx.

The second thing to understand about the spine is the uniqueness of the discs between the bones. They are unlike any other area of the body. They are a thick, mucus-like material encased between the bones but surrounded by a tough layer of crisscrossed rings called the *annulus*. This contained but compressed gel acts as a hydraulic system that can tolerate immense loads and stress. Additionally, the annulus is more similar to a fabric than it is to other joints in the body. And what happens to that Metallica shirt you've been wearing since the mid-90s over time? It fades, attenuates, then finally rips. This is the plague of disc injuries (herniations, bulges, sciatica) you have no doubt heard of or sustained yourself.

Aside from the primary importance of the spine for early embryological development, the spine has the incredible role of surrounding the precious spinal cord and individual nerves as they exit through a host of joints and soft tissue connections. When you take a second to look at the anatomy of the human spine, it almost seems inevitable that Murphy's Law—which states that anything that can go wrong will go wrong—will prove true at some point or another.

Hippocrates intuited the spine's significance more than 2,000 years ago, but even today with the incredible advancements in technology and knowledge, rates of spinal surgeries and complications seem to be endlessly rising. We know its importance, yet we can still underestimate the value of maintaining a healthy spine.

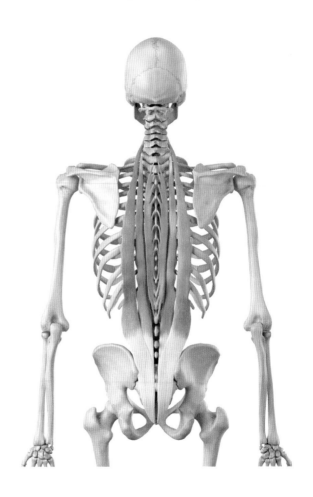

HOW TO GO ABOUT REBUILDING A HEALTHY SPINE

Let's ask ourselves some basic questions. What is the point of the elbow joint? *To bend your arm* (otherwise bars would just be lined with nonplussed patrons staring at full pints in front of them). Since we are not scarecrows, we have joints. What is the fundamental utility of a joint? *To allow movement.* Now, if I explained to you that there are over 100 joints in the human spine alone, what would you say it has evolved to do? *Move.*

Therefore, all the stretches in this chapter are focused on movement of the spine. There are excellent spinal stability exercises that exist in which the primary goal is to *prevent movement* from occurring, and those are sometimes warranted. I would advise you to look up "spine stability exercises" and read about them, as some people are in the equally unenviable position of a spine that moves too much.

If you are someone who moves well and seems quite flexible but are troubled by quick movements or unexpected perturbations (missing a step on a stair, quickly reaching for a falling object, etc.), you may find more value beginning your recovery journey with stability exercises. It can be difficult to discern sometimes on your own, so if ever in doubt, seek professional help for guidance.

Additionally, research has shed light on the benefits of strengthening the spine, particularly via endurance-style training (high-repetition exercises like doing 30 back extensions, or long-duration exercises like planking for a long time) and how it can improve back pain. So, unless contraindicated by your symptoms, essentially everyone may benefit from gaining spinal muscular strength and endurance.

Finding the Right Path Forward

The dual assumption within this book is that not every reader is broken or in pain but rather just needs to avoid continual decay and wants to maintain proper health. The intention of this chapter is to help both. The only caveat is that those in pain may need to be aware that if the upcoming movements make your pain worse, we advise stopping immediately and seeking local professional help.

THE STRETCHES

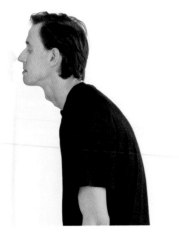

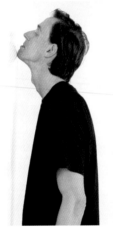

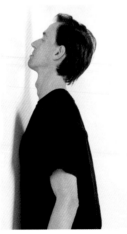

Spinal Waves

Too often people move too much in some areas and not at all in others. When one's connecting bones can move independently of each other, we call this *dissociation*. Here we will focus on dissociation to promote as much intersegmental motion as possible throughout the spine.

Step 1: Stand facing a wall, an inch or two separating your nose from the wall. Lean gently forward until your nose touches.

Step 2: Begin the spinal wave by looking up so that your nose comes off the wall and your chin touches the wall.

Step 3: Continue extending your head until your entire face comes off the wall, but now your upper chest is touching the wall.

Step 4: This wave continues down, bit by bit, as the upper chest comes off but the middle chest touches. Slide all the way down until only the front of the hips are against the wall.

Step 5: At this point the wave reverses. The head tucks downward, followed by the rest of the body, until the body is rounded completely forward and ready to begin again with another wave at Step 1.

Step 6: Repeat for 1 or more minutes. As you improve and the rhythm becomes ingrained, you will no longer need a wall.

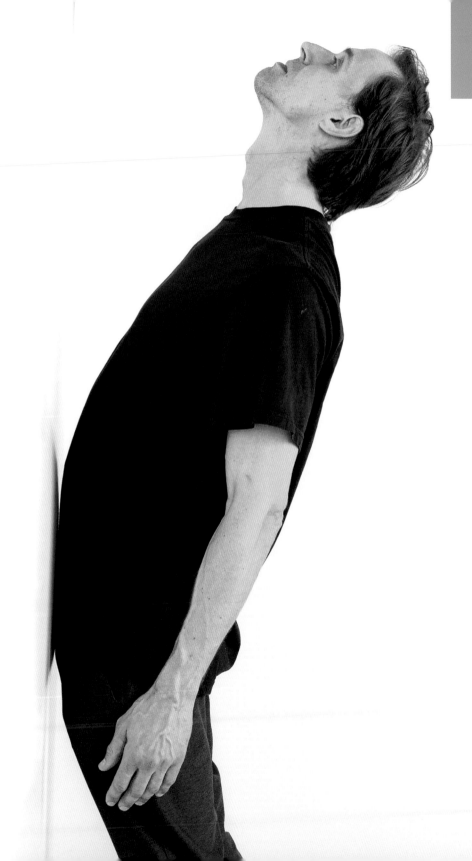

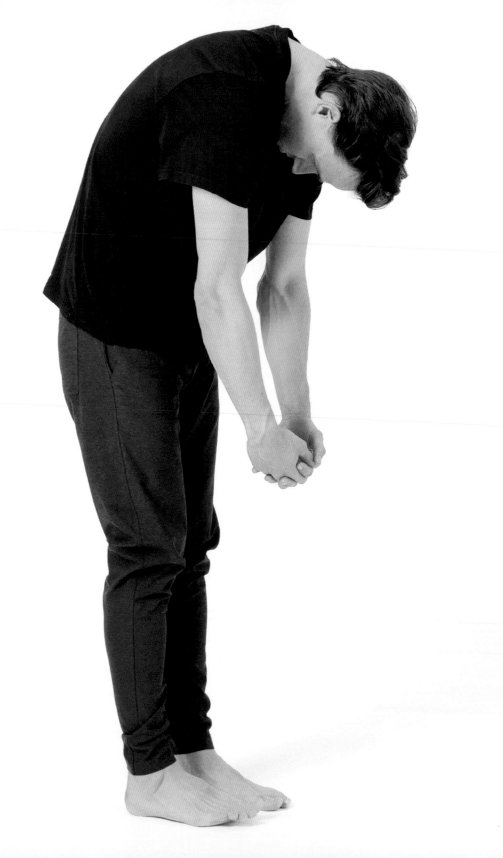

2

Jefferson Curl

This stretch will promote stability and control during a toe touch. Being able to do a fluid, full-range-of-motion Jefferson curl demonstrates hamstring flexibility and strength, pelvic mobility and spinal flexibility as well as balance and coordination.

Step 1: Stand, knees straight, with your hands clasped in front of you as if you were holding a weight in your hands.

Step 2: Try to maintain your hips over your ankles, and avoid shifting your hips back behind your feet as you do the movement. Start by tucking the chin and, therefore, bending the neck forward.

Step 3: It may seem impossible at first, but try to imagine bending just one bone at a time, rolling the spine toward the floor.

Step 4: Continue as far as you can with straight knees. Try to take *no less than 10 seconds* to achieve this.

Step 5: Just gently unlock your knees, and continue a little farther down if your body allows.

Step 6: Once you have your end range there, hold this position and take 2 to 3 deep breaths in through the nose and out through the mouth.

Step 7: Reverse the wave, this time trying to straighten everything from the bottom up. Extend the hips, then the low back, midsection and so forth until you reach the starting position again.

Step 8: Repeat 3 to 5 times.

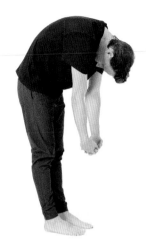

3

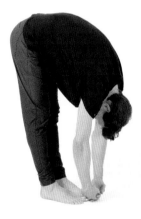

4

Note: For those of you who cannot tolerate this or for whom it reignites back pain, leg pain and/or sciatica, try stopping this movement for a few weeks before trying again. Also make sure your speed is always controlled.

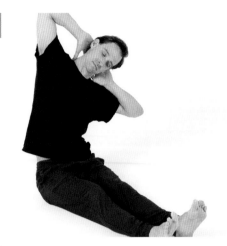

2A

Side Bends (Standing or L-Sit)

The goal here is to acquire the ability to inter-segmentally move the spine side to side. In conjunction with the chapter on thoracic rotation (see page 69), we hammer all directions to promote a healthy spine.

Step 1: You can either stand or L-sit, depending on which position feels better and gives you a deeper stretch.

Step 2: Slowly and under control, attempt to roll the spine down sideways, similarly to the previous spinal wave. Try to avoid bending only at the low back, as most people do with side bends in the gym.

Step 3: Wave yourself back up, starting at the bottom and working your way back to a vertical position.

Step 4: Repeat for 1 or more minutes.

Step 5: Repeat on the other side.

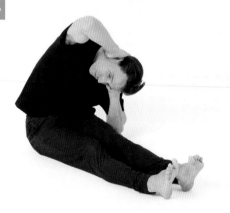

2B

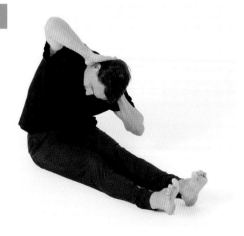

3

MOVING FORWARD

Last but certainly not least, this chapter has hopefully made you painfully aware that the linchpin of the body, the spine, must be cared for. Easily guilty for being the most common malady for humans, we must begin to care for our spines today and not tomorrow.

Research suggests that those most susceptible to spine problems are those who do *too little* (i.e., who work at a desk job and/or do no exercise) and those who do *too much* (e.g., work as a stone-mason). However, as technology and advancements of comfort make living easier, doing too little will continue to be of larger concern. We know of only one true method that works every single time in delaying the degenerative process of aging . . . movement.

"One should first get a knowledge of the structure of the spine; for this is also requisite for many diseases."

—HIPPOCRATES

"For to be free is not merely to cast off one's chains, but to live in a way that respects and enhances the freedom of others."

—NELSON MANDELA

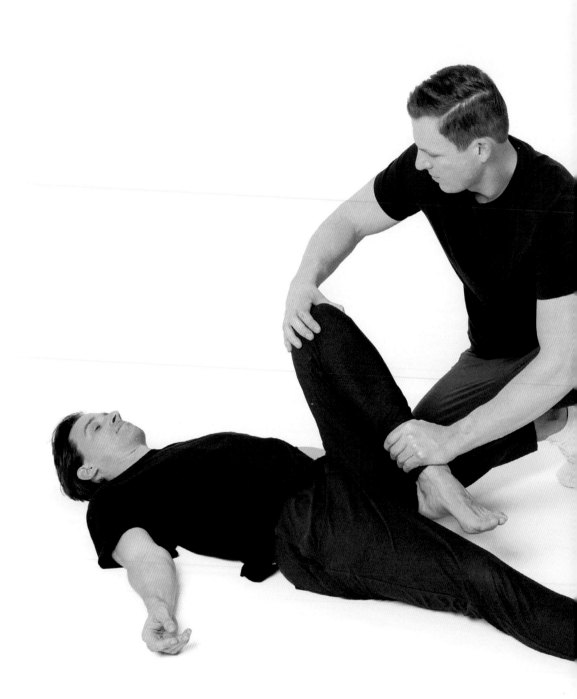

PUTTING IT ALL TOGETHER

Full-Body Integration Movements for Lasting Health

The best endings are beginnings. The exercises and stretches found in this book are meant to be a bridge, not a home. The movements in this chapter are pillars for developing your future self. Just like choosing not to invest is still an investment decision, so is moving. Except an abundance of research shows that choosing to move is one of the best things you can do for your overall health, and that not moving is consistently shown to be harmful to your health. But where should you invest your movement? Let's dive into some basic but powerful movements that focus on moving the eight key areas of the body we went over in this book.

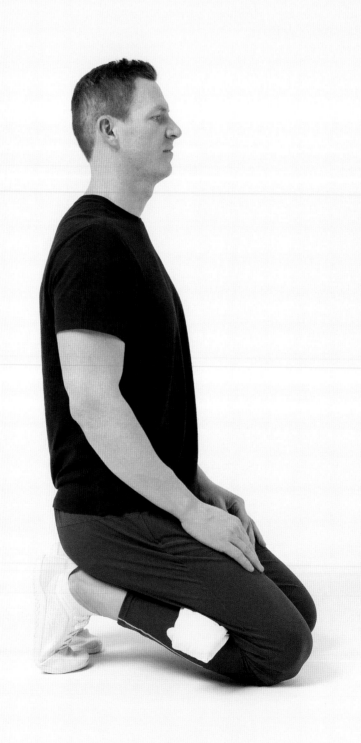

LOOKING FORWARD

The best exercises are the ones you'll do. When people create an exercise regimen, the most common missing piece is play. Golf, pickle ball or slow-pitch softball are workouts disguised as games. Not to mention the mental health benefits of "playing." So, do not substitute the following suggestions for play; both are important. Instead, consider them as attempting to add new dimensions to your body of movement.

The following six movements begin to combine the work you have done in earlier chapters but gently challenge each area to perform at a higher level. Integrating new capacities to your body on a deeper reactive state is the goal. That way, you gain unconscious competence and habituate the hidden potential locked inside you—akin to the skills required to drive a car that have become unconscious actions. This is the secret goal of the movements you'll be learning shortly.

10 Years from Now

Two more overarching ideas to consider as you progress are the weekly frequency at which you do these movements and the extension of your time horizon within each stretch. Dedicating between 30 and 60 minutes three times a week is a realistic goal for having a healthy workout plan. Within these three sessions, you need only do one challenging workout. Leave the other 2 days for light exercise that should leave you feeling better than when you started.

One of the most common reasons patients come to see us is because they have overextended their body beyond their means, and they break down. When you extend your goal to 10 seconds or reps—or as a patient of mine asked, "Why not 50?"—you begin to approach your workouts differently. Without the pressure to produce immediately, you may notice you progress easily.

THE STRETCHES

Squat

Also known as the king of exercises, the squat can be performed in a variety of ways, but you should focus on your speed and load. Initially, you should focus on keeping a consistent speed as you descend into the squat and as you come up from the bottom. But you can also explore what pushing the gas or braking feels like. Pausing at the bottom or going fast down but slow up can vastly change what areas of the body you are targeting during the squat. It is your goal to find what speed gives you the best results.

While the squat movement remains the same, you can add weight to squat in many ways. You should begin with bodyweight, but a goblet squat (weight held in front of your chest like an oversized goblet) and slant board squat (squat normally except start by placing your feet on a board that is slanted downward) are both safe for most people to start with. Traditional squats are great because they allow you to increase the load you move, but because you have 10 years to get strong, you should be in no hurry to add more plates.

Everyone will squat a bit differently, but here are a few tips to make things easier for you. Starting at the bottom, your feet should be a comfortable distance apart. Toes pointing away from each other is easier than toes straight forward. Next, you'll want to fix your gaze on "the horizon" and allow your collarbones to roll upward as your shoulders sink back. Keeping your arms horizontal to the ground is a great guide to knowing if you have a good position in your torso. The chest will be upright, but you will be tilting forward a little. Allow the knees to bend over the toes, and keep your hips back as if you were about to sit down onto a small stool that is just behind your heels.

This is only a guide. If, as you are squatting, you feel you need to make certain changes, you should listen to that intuition. Exercising is a great way to strengthen not only your body but also your intuition.

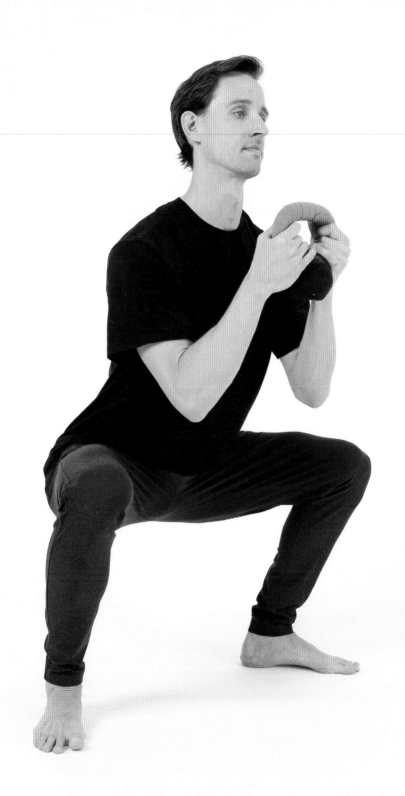

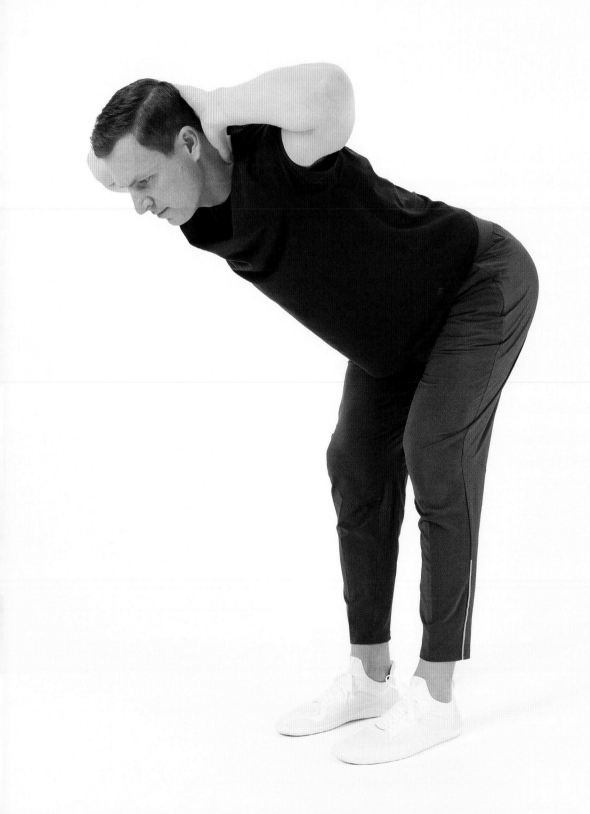

Hinge

Toe touches, sun salutations, good mornings and deadlifts are all hinge-based movements, as they center around the femur and pelvis without the knee bend you see in a squat. The photo to the left illuminates this. While toe touches are the easiest, you may find more benefit in doing this movement with more repetition. The goal with a proper hinge is to sense the posterior chain (glutes and hamstrings) bearing the most tension through the movement. If you notice your back engaging, that is not bad, but try to shift your hips back as if you are closing a car door. This will shift the pressure into the legs and hips, not the back. Training yourself to properly bend at the hips and strengthening your hamstrings may be the number one way to maintain a healthy low back and knee.

Carry

The secret to stable shoulders that don't snap, crackle and pop are carries. A stable shoulder is a strong shoulder. Carries, also known as suitcase carries or farmer's walks, are the first line of defense in repairing rotator cuffs. Your rotator cuff engages when you squeeze and grip something. So, by doing carries, you can target your rotator cuff in a safe way without going through movements that may trigger your shoulder pain. You can also add a lot of load to your carries, which will help strengthen your rotator cuff while minimizing the risk of hurting yourself. The goal is to hold the weight until your grip fails. Then, each time thereafter, your goal is to go a little bit longer.

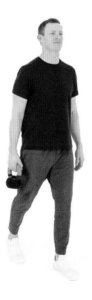
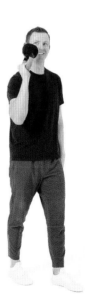

Throw

Throwing is one of the most natural movements. Without being told, you were able to throw as a baby. This movement introduces the idea of building a skill. You are building new skills throughout this entire book, but this may be the most obvious. Having said that, if you are not a thrower by nature, then remind yourself of your 10-year plan. This skill is also beginning to build elasticity into your muscles and joints. There are some who consider this the only real way to get your muscles and joints to adapt. Creating elasticity, bounciness, fluidity and springiness in your body is something you can use with all your movements.

Walk

Walking 5,000 steps a day has been proven to be one of the most consistently beneficial exercises for your overall health. Light cardio has long-lasting benefits. You don't need a gym membership or any fancy techniques for this one. But as you walk, you can focus on a few things. First, it's okay to heel strike (see photo) when walking. Second, you need to feel the "inside edge" of your foot just like in golf or when skiing. Third, keeping your chest up begins with keeping your chin up. Fourth, longer strides are not better. If you notice aches or pains as you walk, shorten your stride. Fifth, swing your arms. Whether you want to imagine pulling a rope or making sure your elbows swing back just a bit, you need to swing your arms when you walk. Walking is a wonderful way to experience the world around you and sneak in some exercise while you're at it.

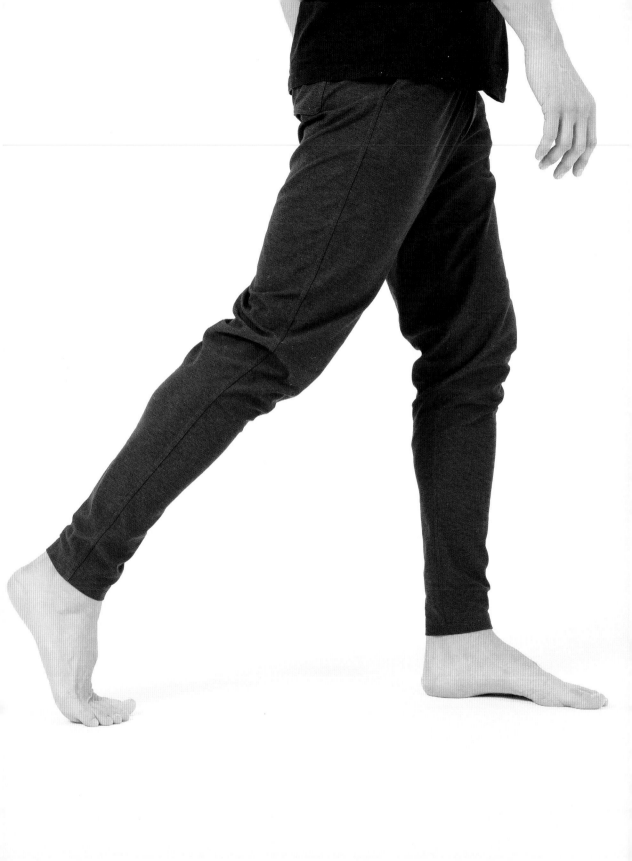

Jump

The skill of jumping rope combines everything you have learned in this book. Building skill, endurance, the stretch reflex and overall strength can be done in just 3 minutes. The goal is to be able to jump rope for 3 minutes. If you can jump rope for 3 minutes, there will be very few things that will challenge you physically in your day-to-day. The end goal is to be able to do all the things life has for you without letting your body get in the way.

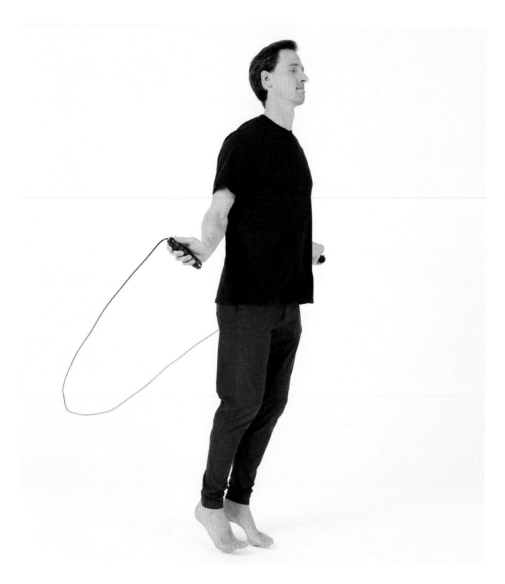

MOVING FORWARD

The aforementioned movements (squat, hinge, jump, etc.), in reality, are our modern attempts to label movement concepts. Doing so gives us a guideline to follow at the gym and lets us categorize movement capacities into things we can understand. This is done not because it is the most optimal way to think about human movement, but rather because it is a convenient way for us to internalize our options.

Throughout history and the evolution of the human species, movement was always a blend of all these things. We might have had to pick up and carry the deer that we had chased for many miles before finally hitting the mark with a finely aimed spear throw and then squat down to build a fire for later that evening. We didn't label things hinge, carry, throw. We simply moved to accomplish a task. The closest thing to this now, if you are not an agrarian or member of a hunter-gatherer tribe, is dynamic sport. Sports such as football and tennis require reaction in a variety of ways that demand the full integration of human movement. The physical therapist Gray Cook stated, "First move well, then move often." This book is an attempt to allow the body access to move well, but don't forget to move often.

"I want to live my life taking the risk—all the time—that I don't know anything like enough yet, that I haven't understood enough, that I can't know enough, that I'm always hungrily operating on the margins of a potentially great harvest of future knowledge and wisdom . . . . Take the risk of thinking for yourself; much more happiness, truth, beauty and wisdom will come to you."

–CHRISTOPHER HITCHENS

ANATOMY CHART

Muscular System

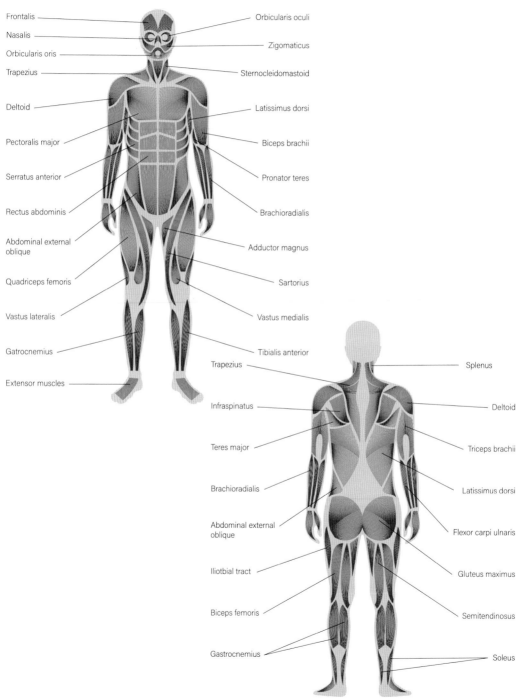

Frontalis

Nasalis

Orbicularis oris

Trapezius

Deltoid

Pectoralis major

Serratus anterior

Rectus abdominis

Abdominal external oblique

Quadriceps femoris

Vastus lateralis

Gatrocnemius

Extensor muscles

Orbicularis oculi

Zigomaticus

Sternocleidomastoid

Latissimus dorsi

Biceps brachii

Pronator teres

Brachioradialis

Adductor magnus

Sartorius

Vastus medialis

Tibialis anterior

Trapezius

Infraspinatus

Teres major

Brachioradialis

Abdominal external oblique

Iliotbial tract

Biceps femoris

Gastrocnemius

Splenus

Deltoid

Triceps brachii

Latissimus dorsi

Flexor carpi ulnaris

Gluteus maximus

Semitendinosus

Soleus

Skeletal System

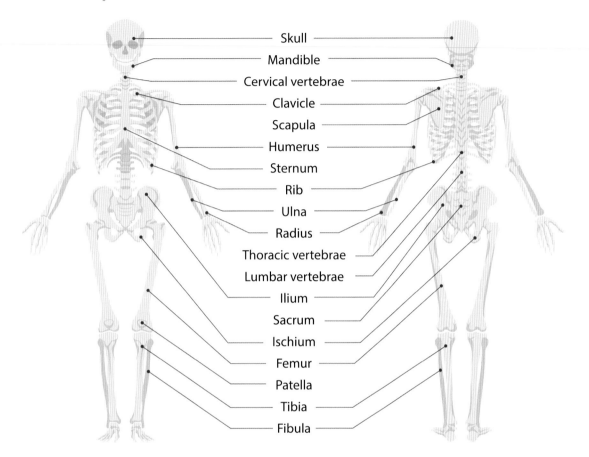

Skull

Mandible

Cervical vertebrae

Clavicle

Scapula

Humerus

Sternum

Rib

Ulna

Radius

Thoracic vertebrae

Lumbar vertebrae

Ilium

Sacrum

Ischium

Femur

Patella

Tibia

Fibula

ACKNOWLEDGMENTS

The book before you would not have been possible without the following people:

My coauthor and friend John Cybulski, who agreed to head down this crazy road with me years ago. An inspired road cloaked in uncertainty. One adorned with hundreds of podcasts, thousands of texts, facilitated by Belgian tripels and accompanied by a commensurate yearning for knowledge.

My patients through the years, who make me better and perennially remind me that I don't know anything like enough yet.

Our editor at Page Street, Franny Donington, who saw something in us besides a social media following and helped us create something that would have otherwise been quite possibly unreadable.

My family and friends. For making me a lover of books. A lover of learning.

My wife, who, without request and often undeserved, continually goes out of her way in search of ways to support me.

And my son, Soren, the constant reminder of my mortality and vulnerability, my ultimate impetus to stay healthy, to stay . . . alive.

—BLR

This book has been made possible by the support and love of my beautiful, patient and gracious wife, Jessica. And by my coworkers, colleagues and patients over the years who taught me how to listen and learn.

—JTC

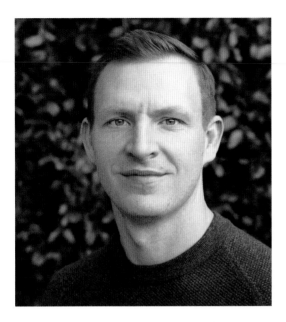

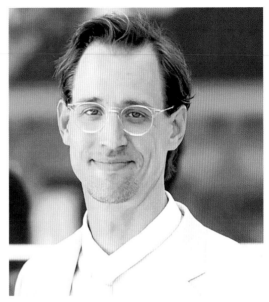

Bobby Riley holds a doctorate in chiropractic from Northwestern Health Sciences University in Minnesota. He was a ten-time All-American and three-time National Champion in track and field at the University of Wisconsin–La Crosse, where he completed his undergraduate studies. He has practiced rehabilitation-focused chiropractic for over ten years, in the U.S.A., Iceland and the Netherlands. He has worked with hundreds of professional athletes and is the co-owner of The Anatomy of Therapy, which has over a million followers.

John Cybulski earned his doctorate in chiropractic from Texas Chiropractic College in 2010 after playing college soccer at West Texas A&M. After practicing in Central Texas for over a decade, he founded The Anatomy of Therapy, which receives between two and ten million views per month. He now lives in Los Angeles, California, with his wife, Jessica. Having recently settled in LA, he maintains his chiropractic practice as well as creates content for social media, writing and podcasting. In his free time, he enjoys exploring the great outdoors, working out and hanging out with friends and family.

Reverse Nordic Curls, 43, 47

Reverse Nordic Curl Variation, 44

rotation and, 25, 35, 37, 44, 47, 51

squats, 108

Tailor's Pose, 20

Tall Kneeling to Child's Pose Sitting, 44

tibia, 36

torque, 13, 37, 46, 47

Towel Bends, 40

Towel Bend Variations, 41

triggers, 35

L

latissimus dorsi muscle, 116

ligaments, 25, 36

locomotion, 51, 93

low back pain

    adductor (groin) and, 17

    bipedalism and, 93

    costs of, 12, 93

    effort and, 62

    hinge and, 111

    hips and, 52, 59, 61, 62

    Reverse Nordic Curls and, 43

    stretch stress and, 62

lumbar vertebrae, 117

M

Mandela, Nelson, 103

mandible, 117

mechanotransduction, 82, 84

meniscus, 36

Michener, James, 47

muscles

    abdominal external oblique, 116

    adductor brevis, 17

    adductor longus, 17

    adductor magnus, 17

    biceps brachii, 116

    biceps femoris, 116

    brachioradialis, 116

    deltoid, 116

    exhalation muscles, 74

    extensor muscles, 116

    flexor carpi ulnaris, 116

    frontalis, 116

    gastrocnemius, 116

    gluteus maximus, 116

    gracilis, 17

    hamstring, 36, 111

    iliotibial band, 38, 116

    infraspinatus, 116

    inhalation muscles, 74

    latissimus dorsi, 116

    nasalis, 116

    orbicularis oris, 116

    pectineus, 17

    pectoralis major, 116

    quadriceps, 36, 116

    rectus abdominis, 116

    rectus femoris, 38

    sartorius, 38, 116

    semitendinosus, 116

    serratus anterior, 116

    soleus, 116

    splenius capitis, 116

    supraspinatus, 83

    teres major, 116

    throwing and, 112

    trapezius, 116

    triceps brachii, 116

    vastus lateralis, 38, 116

    vastus medialis, 38, 116

    zygomaticus, 116

N

nasalis muscle, 116

O

orbicularis oris muscle, 116

orcas, 91

osteoarthritis, 83

over-pronation, 25, 26

P

pain

    adductor (groin) health and, 17

    adhesive capsulitis, 83

    back, 12, 17, 43, 52, 59, 61, 62, 67, 71–73, 93, 95–97, 111

    bipedalism and, 93

    breathing, 73

    clues to, 72

    costs of, 12, 93

    disc injuries, 95

    dislocations, 83

    foot, 27

    frozen shoulder, 83

    hinge and, 111

    hips, 49, 52, 53, 59, 61, 62

    knees, 25, 35, 39, 40

    knots, 72

    load capacity and, 39

    low back, 12, 17, 43, 52, 59, 61, 62, 93

    osteoarthritis, 83